Alcohol,
   Other Drugs
      and Violent Death

Alcohol, Other Drugs and Violent Death

Paul W. Haberman

Senior Research Associate
Center for Socio-Cultural Research on Drug Use
School of Public Health, Columbia University

Michael M. Baden, M.D.

Deputy Chief Medical Examiner, City of New York
Associate Professor of Forensic Medicine, New York University
Adjunct Professor of Law, New York Law School
Visiting Professor of Pathology, Albert Einstein School of Medicine

New York
OXFORD UNIVERSITY PRESS
1978

To Elinor, Matthew, and Karen
and
To Judi, Trissa, Judson, Lindsey, and Sarah.

Library of Congress Cataloging in Publication Data

Haberman, Paul W., 1928–
  Alcohol, other drugs, and violent death.

  Bibliography: p.
  Includes index.
  1. Alcoholism—New York (City)   2. Drug abuse—New York (City)   3. Violent
deaths—New York (City)   4. Death—Causes.   I. Baden, Michael M., joint author.
II. Title.—[DNLM: 1. Alcoholism.   2. Drug   abuse.   3. Homicide—Violence—Accidents.   WM274.3   H114a]   HV5298.N5H3   362.2'9'097471   78-2752   ISBN
0-19-502359-5

Printed in the United States of America

Preface

The role of alcohol and other drugs in fatal accidents, homicides, and suicides has been described. Studies of the association between substance abuse and violent death have typically dealt with each relationship separately, alcohol and motor vehicle accidents, in particular. The major purpose of this book is to present a more detailed, interdisciplinary analysis of these various relationships in the same large urban area. This approach is made possible by the large amount of data collected, in terms of both the number of cases for each violent cause of death and the amount of relevant information on the dead persons and the circumstances of death.

There are in our study more than 500 homicide victims, 300 suicides, about 400 who were fatally injured in motor vehicle or other accidents, and over 600 who died directly of alcoholism and/or narcotism. Among the 1,954 sample cases, almost 600 were identified as alcoholics, over 300 as narcotics abusers, and some 200 as having both conditions. Evidence for these classifications was drawn both from informants and postmortem physical examinations. Other studies of violent death and drug use have usually involved fewer cases and less data. Most often they have been drawn retrospectively from only one source of information, such as death certificates, and the analysis of cases has usually been less extensive.

Our major sources of original Medical Examiner data were a questionnaire given in person to study informants when they identified the decedents at the Office of Chief Medical Examiner in New York City and concurrent autopsy and toxicologic findings. Other Medical Examiner and Police Department data on homicide motives, victim-perpetrator relationships, and fatal traffic accidents were also utilized.

Drinking and drug problems among decedents are often denied by informants, knowingly or not, and they are not always revealed in postmortem physical findings. The availability of Medical Examiner data on alcohol and narcotics abuse that was collected systematically from several sources gave us a unique opportunity to determine the nature and extent to which these problems were underestimated.

Multiple use or abuse of mood-altering substances, including alcohol, is a rather common occurrence of growing interest to re-searchers. In our sample, we have analyzed in detail the association between violent death and different patterns of multiple drug use, primarily alcohol and/or narcotics used in combination with other depressants such as barbiturates and tranquilizers.

Some evidence that alcoholism, narcotism, and nonspecific substance abuse tend to occur in families has been published. Not very much, however, has been reported to date on the possible relationship between this familial tendency and unnatural deaths. For this reason we collected data about the cause of death and drinking or drug problems of close relatives of decedents—spouses, parents, siblings, and children—to investigate such familial patterns of substance abuse in conjunction with unnatural deaths.

Various attempts have been made to use mortality data to estimate the prevalence of alcoholism and narcotism. In this book we have proposed new methods of utilizing Medical Examiner data for this purpose and for insight into trends in substance abuse.

The book, then, is about alcohol and narcotics abuse among adults who died unnaturally in New York City—the largest urban Medical Examiner population in the world—during a one-year period. Among the major findings are the extent to which alcohol and narcotics abuse are involved in homicides, suicides, and fatal accidents, the interrelationship of problems with both alcohol and other drugs in unnatural deaths, and the underreporting of substance abuse as the most common underlying factor in such deaths.

April 1978   P.W.H.
                                                                    M.M.B.

Acknowledgments

The study reported in this book would not have been possible without the cooperation of the Chief Medical Examiner of the City of New York, Dr. Dominick J. DiMaio, and the staff of the Medical Examiner's Office. Dr. Jack Elinson and Dr. Eric Josephson at the Center for Socio-Cultural Research on Drug Use, Columbia University, provided advice and resources throughout the project. Many useful recommendations were also made by other colleagues at the Center. Jeffrey W. House, our editor at Oxford University Press, gave us very sound advice and criticism throughout. The format reflects his fine judgment.

Special thanks are due to the project personnel who carried out their assignments conscientiously and efficiently. Eileen D. Schuster had the primary responsibility for interviewing informants and obtaining relevant medical findings on the sample cases, assisted by Betsy Feldman. Phyllis Starner capably handled administrative and research details while the data were being collected, processed, tabulated, and analyzed. Ms. Schuster, Ms. Starner, and Jane A. Ungemack all made constructive editorial suggestions. Marilyn J. Mara produced several typed drafts of the manuscript from barely legible handwritten copy, with the assistance of Estelle Kirsh.

The help of others is greatly appreciated. Dr. James C. Teegarden of the National Institute on Alcohol Abuse and Alcoholism encouraged this work. Jeffrey A. Starr and programmers at Datatab, Inc.

produced the essential cross-tabulations and other computer output. The New York City Police Department generously provided additional data on homicides and fatal traffic accidents. Sgt. Henry G. Schaaff and the staff in the Crime Analysis Section assisted us in obtaining information on more than 500 homicides. Sgt. Frank Ghiorsi, in the Vehicle Homicide Investigations Section, compiled the details on selected traffic fatalities.

This study was supported primarily by a National Institute on Alcohol Abuse and Alcoholism Grant (2-RO1-AA-00303) to Columbia University; additional support was provided by the Center for Socio-Cultural Research on Drug Use, Columbia University (National Institute on Drug Abuse Grant 5-PO1-DA-01097).

Contents

1

Highlights of the Study

Background

In New York City, the Office of the Chief Medical Examiner investigates all sudden, medically unattended, traumatic, unusual, or suspicious deaths, including all suspected homicides, suicides, accidents, and narcotics-related deaths. All deaths due to acute alcoholism and associated with chronic alcoholism when trauma is a possible factor in the death must also be reported to the Medical Examiner's Office. Every such death occurring in four of the five city boroughs — excluding Brooklyn — was investigated at the Medical Examiner's Office in Manhattan when this study was being conducted.

The sample for our study consisted of 1954 persons eighteen years of age or older who were thought to have died unnaturally when initially seen at the Medical Examiner's Office and who were identified by relatives or other informants at that office during the twelve months from August 20, 1974 to August 19, 1975. It was subsequently determined that nearly all died as a result of homicide, suicide, accident, alcoholism, narcotism, or acute drug poisoning. The study sample comprises 3 to 4 percent of all adults who died in the Bronx, Manhattan, Queens, and Staten Island and about one-half of all unnatural deaths investigated by the Medical Examiner's Office during the twelve-month study period.

1

Sixty-five percent of the sample cases were less than 45 years old, 76 percent were men, and 59 percent were nonwhite. These cases, like the New York City medical examiner population in general, are predominantly black or Hispanic men, less than 45 years of age who lived and died in Manhattan. The sample is representative of the total medical examiner population during the study year in the same age and cause-of-death categories. By contrast, the adult population of New York City is older, mostly white, and 55 percent are women.

Classifying Decedents as Alcoholics and Narcotics Abusers

Decedents were classified as alcoholics and narcotics abusers on the basis of informant reports or physical findings of related problems. Informant classification of decedents as alcoholics was based on responses to questions about any health problems ever and any family, money, job, or other problems ever because of drinking. Informant classification of decedents as narcotics abusers was based on responses to questions about any problems ever because of narcotics use.

Physical classification of decedents as alcoholics was based on the certification of the cause of death as acute and/or chronic alcoholism alone or in conjunction with another cause, or an autopsy finding that could almost always be attributed to alcoholism in this medical examiner population. These postmortem findings are moderate or severe fatty change in the liver, cirrhosis of the liver, and, rarely, pancreatitis or ruptured esophageal varices unrelated to another disease or condition. (Among persons under medical care, these postmortem findings more than one time in ten may be related to some disease or condition other than alcoholism.) Physical classification of decedents as narcotics abusers was based on the certification of the cause of death as acute and/or chronic narcotism alone or with another cause, or on toxicologic findings of morphine (the heroin metabolite), methadone, or adulterants for heroin, with narcotics use implicated by needle marks or elsewhere in the case history.

Fifty-eight percent of the 1954 sample cases had an identified problem with alcohol, narcotics, or both; 41 percent were classified as alcoholics and 28 percent as narcotics abusers. The specific proportions are: alcoholics 30 percent; narcotics abusers 17 percent; both conditions 11 percent; and neither condition 42 percent.

Only 17 percent of the 803 alcoholics and 20 percent of the narcotics abusers were classified as such by informants alone without physical evidence. Larger proportions — 44 percent of the alcoholics and 29 percent of the narcotics abusers — were classified only on the basis of physical evidence without informant affirmation. The remainder — 39 percent of the alcoholics and 51 percent of the narcotics abusers — had both informant and physical evidence of problems related to the abuse of alcohol or narcotics.

Physical evidence in most cases included cause-of-death certification of alcoholism and/or narcotism. Fifty-five percent of the narcotics abusers were classified as such on the basis of cause-of-death certification; 24 percent were so classified on the basis of toxicologic findings of morphine or methadone with some other cause of death. Forty-six percent of the alcoholics had their cause of death certified as alcoholism; 37 percent were classified as such on the basis of autopsy findings, primarily liver damage due to alcohol use, and officially there was another cause of death.

The physical findings used to classify decedents as alcoholics — mainly autopsy evidence of liver damage — are a manifestation of chronic alcoholism, whereas toxicologic findings used to classify decedents as narcotics abusers are an indication of recent use of heroin or methadone and probably of an acute reaction. Chronic abuse was indicated for most of the 370 persons whose cause of death included alcoholism, while acute (intravenous) narcotism was indicated for most of the 307 narcotics abusers who died of this cause.

The blood or brain alcohol concentration (BAC) for 13 percent of persons who died of alcoholism was 0.30 percent or higher, which makes death from acute alcoholism alone a possibility. Because alcohol is metabolized by the body at a rate of approximately 0.015 percent per hour, a larger proportion undoubtedly had peak concentrations this high some time shortly before death.

Fifty-three percent of the 239 persons reported to be heavy drinkers without any related problems were classified as alcoholics by physical evidence, confirming the likelihood of unreported problems because of drinking. Twenty percent were narcotics abusers without any evidence of alcoholism observable by our study methods. Much of the denial of problems caused by heavy drinking in our study may result from a lack of strong sanctions against alcoholism in some sociocultural groups and from the low socioeconomic status resulting in other social problems irrespective of drinking problems.

Most of the decedents were identified by a close relative—sibling, spouse, parent, or child. Children were more likely to be informants for alcoholics, and parents were more often informants for narcotics abusers, which reflects the considerable age difference at the time of death between alcoholics and narcotics abusers. Fifty-four percent of the alcoholics were 40 years of age or older; 60 percent of the narcotics abusers were less than 30.

Although no particular relative was more or less likely to acknowledge the decedents' alcoholism or narcotism, there seemed to be real differences in admission or denial of alcohol or narcotics problems according to closeness of informants and decedents. Alcoholics who last spoke to the informants within one day of their death were more often classified as alcoholics by physical evidence alone rather than by informants. But narcotics abusers with the same proximity to informants were more often classified as such by the informants rather than by physical evidence alone. Similarly, when questioned about the 222 decedents having both conditions, 46 percent of the informants denied the decedents' alcoholism, but only 22 percent denied their narcotism.

The greater denial by informants of alcoholism among decedents than of narcotism might be explained in part by: (a) the legality of alcoholic beverages, the relatively slow progression of alcoholism, and the tolerance or presence of heavy social drinking or incipient problem drinking in the alcoholic's family; and (b) the illegality, high cost, and relatively rapid addictive properties of narcotics.

While alcohol and other drugs have an appreciable contributory role in suicides, homicides, and fatal accidents, substance abuse itself was by far the major cause of death among study cases classified as alcoholics, narcotics abusers, or both. Forty-seven percent of the alcoholics died of alcoholism; 55 percent of the narcotics abusers died of narcotism; and in 72 percent of those with both conditions the cause of death was due to abuse of one or both substances.

There was a considerable amount of underreporting by informants in our study of problems due to alcohol or narcotics use. By contrast, in a smaller, but not inconsequential number of cases there was no physical evidence of reported problems. Forty-five percent of the alcoholics and 29 percent of the narcotics abusers were classified by physical evidence only, and about one-fifth in each subgroup were classified by informants alone. Thus despite the large proportions whose cause of death was directly attributable to substance abuse, a sizeable minority of our cases would not have been classified as alcoholics or narcotics abusers if only one case-finding method had been used.

Multiple Drug Abuse

Depressants such as alcohol, narcotics, sedatives, and tranquilizers are more life-threatening than other groups of mood-altering substances such as stimulants or hallucinogens. Multiple drug use among our medical examiner cases consists primarily of concomitant use of depressants; positive findings of concomitant use of different substances can be determined by means of toxicologic tests, but sequential use is not likely to be revealed due to the time span between the use of different substances.

Toxicologic findings were obtained for 1429 persons, 73 percent of the total sample. The 525 cases for which toxicologic tests were not considered necessary are excluded from most of the findings in this section.

Informants were likely to report the decedents' drug of choice as the cause of related problems, suggesting chronic abuse. Twenty-eight percent were reported to have had some problem because of drug use, with multiple use indicated in 8 percent of the cases. Heroin was mentioned by 20 percent of the informants — much more often than any other drug. Barbiturates (6%) and illicitly used methadone (2%) were the only other drugs mentioned by more than 1 percent of the informants. It can not be determined whether methadone use reported for patients in treatment programs included illicit as well as treatment doses, so that more than 2 percent probably had problems due to illicit methadone use.

Positive toxicologic findings in our sample generally indicated recent use before death by chronic abusers of their drug of choice and/or substitutes. However, a few decedents with toxicologic evidence of recent drug use were only occasional users or experimenters—or had used pills to commit suicide. Forty-two percent of the decedents on whom toxicologic tests were performed had used some mood-altering substance shortly before death, including multiple use in 17 percent of the cases. Methadone (17%), morphine (13%), tranquilizers (12%), and barbiturates (12%) were the drugs most often present in toxicologic tests. Morphine was most frequently found alone (7%), but methadone was most often used concomitantly with non-narcotic drugs (10%). Concomitant use of heroin and methadone occurred in 4 percent of the cases. Seventy-one percent of the decedents classified by informants as narcotics abusers showed toxicologic evidence of recent narcotics use, and 73 percent of those reported to have had no drug problems had no postmortem evidence of drug use.

Positive BACs were most common among alcoholics (63%), followed by those with both conditions (51%), nonabusers (33%), and narcotics abusers (25%). A majority with positive BACs in all these subgroups except for narcotics abusers had concentrations of 0.10 percent or above which indicates impairment or intoxication. Alcholics were most likely to have used alcohol and nonnarcotic drugs concomitantly (13%). A substantial percentage of nonabusers who took mood-altering drugs before death were suicide victims, primarily by an overdose of pills.

Among all narcotics abusers in our study, methadone (49%) was found in toxicologic tests more often than morphine (37%). Comparable proportions had postmortem evidence of alcohol use in combination with methadone (14%) or morphine (12%) and concomitant use of both these narcotics (11%).

Deaths attributed to heroin have often been mislabeled as being caused by "overdose" when in fact many of these deaths are due to acute reactions to adulterants of the heroin, the unsterile manner in which it is taken, and possibly multiple drug abuse. Deaths related to methadone use, however, are often due to true pharmacological overdose by persons who obtain illicit methadone, predissolved in juice, which may contain up to 20 times more narcotics than a packet of "street" heroin does. Toxicologic findings in our study indicate concomitant use of alcohol and/or other mood-altering drugs in many deaths attributed to narcotism. One-half of the 226 cases whose cause of death was narcotism had toxicologic evidence of both narcotics and other mood-altering substances. Methadone was present in about twice as many cases as morphine, both alone and in combination with alcohol and/or other drugs. Sixteen percent had evidence of both heroin and methadone use just before death.

The evidence of widespead use of heroin by narcotics abusers who were reported to be patients in a Methadone Maintenance Treatment Program (MMTP) and use of illicit methadone by reported nonpatients in our study sample is striking. Thirty-one percent of 219 MMTP patients and 33 percent of 112 nonpatients had toxicologic evidence of morphine. Methadone was found in 54 percent of the patients and 43 percent of the nonpatients. Patients, presumably stabilized on methadone, may also take heroin. However, it is not now possible to determine the extent to which postmortem findings of methadone exceeded patients' maintenance treatment doses.

Of the 217 cases in which methadone was present at death including deaths due to trauma and to drug-taking directly, 46 percent were nonpatients, 23 percent were previous patients, and 31 percent were current patients. The nonpatients and previous patients were using methadone illicitly and many current patients may have taken more than their daily maintenance doses.

In demographic terms, the decedents classified as alcoholics differed markedly from the narcotics abusers and from those with both conditions. Those with both conditions resembled the narcotics abusers, differing from them mainly in that they were older and apparently were almost all primarily narcotics abusers who also abused alcohol rather than alcoholics who had become narcotics addicts. Those with both conditions showed evidence of physical damage due to alcohol abuse almost as often as alcoholics did. There was physical evidence of alcoholism in 86 percent of 506 autopsied alcoholics and in 76 percent of 207 autopsied persons who had both conditions.

Our data did not demonstrate any increase in narcotics users as a result of the reported widespread use of heroin among American soldiers in Vietnam in 1970–71. Vietnam War veterans comprise 15 percent of the narcotics abusers in our sample and 10 percent of the alcoholics, those with both conditions, and the nonabusers who were men eligible for service then. A larger proportion, about 22 percent of all service-age men living in New York City were Vietnam veterans. Moreover, the Vietnam veterans were in the age, ethnic, and socio-economic groups most vulnerable to heroin addiction; lived in an area where illicit drugs were relatively easy to obtain; and appeared to be similar to our nonveteran addicts.

Suicides, Homicides, and Fatal Accidents

Apart from substance abuse, homicide was the leading cause of death of narcotics abusers, alcoholics, and those with both conditions. Thirty-two percent of the narcotics abusers and 18 percent of the alcoholics and those with both conditions were homicide victims. Homicide was the leading cause of death of persons classified as nonabusers.

Of 546 homicide victims in our study, 46 percent were classified as substance abusers. Similarly, 29 percent of all suicides, 28 percent of all motor vehicle fatalities, and 39 percent of other accident victims were alcoholics, narcotics abusers, or both. Chronic alcoholics in particular contributed large proportions to each of these violent death categories—from 18 percent of the suicides to 28 percent of the other accident victims.

Well over half of all homicides of adults in New York City may involve substance abusers as victims, perpetrators, or both. About one-half of all violent deaths are associated with alcohol use, and about the same amount of alcohol use may occur among the offenders in cases of homicide and other fatal violence. Adding to this the medical examiner cases involving narcotics users, at present more than two-thirds of the violent deaths in New York City are associated with the use or abuse of these substances.

Forty-six percent of the 546 homicide victims in our study were killed by friends, acquaintances, or relatives; in 46 percent of our cases the motive was a dispute. Strangers committed 27 percent of the homicides, and the motive in 21 percent was a crime such as robbery. The relationship in 23 percent and the motive in 17 percent of the cases were still unknown six months after the interviews were completed.

More suicide victims than those in other violent death categories, irrespective of their classification as alcoholics, narcotics abusers, or nonabusers, were women and white, and a relatively large proportion were reported to have had symptoms of depression or other mental illness most of the year before their death. More than in other violent death categories, homicide victims, regardless of their classification as substance abusers or nonabusers, were Hispanic or black men who had not graduated from high school.

The most common means of committing suicide used by the 336 victims in our study were jumping from heights and taking an overdose of pills. Fifty-three percent of the homicides and 13 percent of the suicides in our study were committed with guns. Guns are used in about two-thirds of all homicides and in one-half of all suicides in the United States, i.e., use of guns as a murder weapon is only 15 percent higher, but as a suicide weapon is 40 percent higher, nationally than in New York City.

Alcoholics and narcotics abusers who committed suicide were somewhat more likely to use pills, whereas nonabusers tended to jump from heights more often. Guns were a somewhat more common means of murdering narcotics abusers and nonabusers, whereas alcoholics tended to be killed more often by stab wounds or assault. There were about 1.2 suicides for every homicide in the United States in 1974, while in New York City, as reflected in our sample, there were only 0.6 suicides for every homicide.

Among motor vehicle fatalities, the drivers were almost all men, and 46 percent were less than 30 years old. The pedestrians were mostly men and were older than the drivers, 71 percent being 50 years of age or more. Most of the passengers were women with a similar age distribution as the drivers. These sex and age distributions of fatally injured drivers and pedestrians in our study are similar to comparable data gathered elsewhere. As in other mortality data from urban areas, dead pedestrians outnumbered dead drivers.

In the three subgroups of substance abusers, only the alcoholics comprised an appreciable proportion of suicides, motor vehicle fatalities, and other fatal accident victims. About 10 percent of the alcoholics were in each of these cause-of-death categories. The 263 alcoholics in our study who died of chronic alcoholism were more often black and single, and their principal activity frequently seemed to be drinking or doing nothing. The 61 alcoholics who committed suicide were more likely to be white, married, and in the labor force.

The alcoholics were much older than the narcotics abusers, but their ages did not vary much in relation to their cause of death. Among the nonabusers, the homicide and suicide victims tended to be younger than the accident victims. Whether or not they were substance abusers, many of the persons who died as a result of nontraffic accidents were reported to be sick or engaged in nonproductive activities — substance abuse, nothing, or jail — most of the year preceding their death.

Alcohol was used by a larger percentage of victims in all cause-of-death categories than any other mood-altering substance, except for persons who committed suicide by an overdose of pills. More than one-half of the fatally injured motor vehicle drivers and other accident victims had positive BACs; the proportion with alcohol levels of 0.10 percent or more ranged from 38 percent of the drivers to 53 percent of the drowning victims. Forty-two percent of the homicide victims had some alcohol in their system and 27 percent had levels of at least 0.10 percent. Except for 15 percent of the suicide victims with BACs of 0.01 to 0.09 percent, the comparable percentages for suicide, and pedestrian or motor vehicle passenger fatalities were somewhat smaller.

Non-narcotic drugs — mostly tranquilizers and barbiturates — were detected in toxicologic tests in 86 percent of the suicide victims who had taken pill overdoses, 22 percent of the other suicide victims, 18 percent of the fire victims, and about 10 percent of the other accident fatalities. Narcotics were most often present in homicide victims; 18 percent had toxicologic evidence of recent heroin and/or methadone use.

Familial Drinking and Drug-Use Problems

Fifteen percent of the alcoholics in our study had at least one close relative (parent, sibling, spouse, or child) who was reported to have an alcohol problem, and 9 percent of the narcotics abusers had a relative with a narcotics problem. For those with both conditions, the percentages of reported problems among close relatives were alcoholism 13 percent and narcotics abuse 10 percent.

Informants who denied that decedents had a drinking or drug problem were more likely to deny such problems among close relatives of the deceased than were informants who acknowledged decedents' alcoholism or narcotism. Decedents classified as alcoholics or narcotics abusers by informants were three times more likely to have close relatives reported to be substance abusers than were alcoholics or narcotics abusers classified by physical evidence alone.

The percentage of all alcoholics and narcotics abusers having close relatives with comparable problems can be estimated at 20 percent or more. Our familial rates of alcoholism or narcotism would then be approximately three and ten times the estimated overall prevalence rates of 7 and 2 percent, respectively, indicating that both are familial conditions with an environmental and/or genetic etiology.

Seventy-nine percent of all decedents classified as alcoholics in our study were men. Similarly 61 siblings of 49 alcoholic decedents were reported to have a drinking problem and 74 percent of them were brothers. But as more women drink and as they drink more, a larger percentage will be at risk of having related problems and of becoming alcoholics.

Among the parents of narcotics abusers in our sample, alcohol was almost always implicated as the drug which caused problems, strongly suggesting a change over time in substance abuse away from reliance on alcohol alone to heroin. Multiple drug use in our sample indicates that a relatively large proportion of the decedents had problems related to both narcotics and alcohol use, and that currently a variety of drugs may be found in postmortem toxicologic tests on narcotics abusers and alcoholics. Based on our data, homicide and suicide also run in families. Homicide was the most frequent mode of violent death among close relatives of our sample cases. Close relatives most often died in the same violent manner as persons in our sample.

2

Background

Office of Chief Medical Examiner, New York City

New York City, with a population of almost 8,000,000, has approximately 80,000 deaths annually. Some 30,000 in each recent year have been investigated by the Office of Chief Medical Examiner, and in about one-half of these cases, the death certificate is issued at the scene of death, and the body is not removed to a borough mortuary.

All medically unattended, sudden, traumatic, unusual, or suspicious deaths in New York City are investigated by the Office of Chief Medical Examiner; these include all suspected homicides, suicides, fatal accidents, or narcotics-related deaths. Every death of this kind occurring in four of the five city boroughs—excluding Brooklyn— was investigated at the Medical Examiner's Office in Manhattan while this study was underway. Brooklyn cases were investigated in the Brooklyn office. Homicides, suicides, and fatal accidents are characterized as violent deaths, whereas those due to narcotism or alcoholism are considered unnatural and in a classification by themselves.

When our study was being done, cases from the Bronx, Queens, and Staten Island that required autopsies were brought to the Medical Examiner's Office in Manhattan for identification and postmortem examination. Cases that do not require autopsy can be identified and certified at the individual borough mortuaries. During the study, certificates were issued less often at the scene for medical examiner cases who died in Manhattan and did not require an autopsy than for those who died in the other boroughs. Consequently, autopsies were performed on a smaller porportion of persons who died in Manhattan than on those who died in the Bronx, Queens, and Staten Island. Approximately 8000 autopsies are performed every year at this Medical Examiner's Office.

All deaths due to acute alcoholism and all those associated with chronic alcoholism when trauma is a possible factor in the death must be reported to the Medical Examiner's Office. Deaths of hospitalized patients which are caused by the effects of chronic alcoholism, however, are not always reported. A few cases of alcoholism are also missed because cardiovascular disease has been certified at the scene as the cause of death.

Sample Requirements

We performed a preliminary investigation of the relationships between alcohol, other drugs, and violent death in 1972 (1). The sample for this pilot study consisted of 1000 consecutive cases of decedents eighteen years of age or older identified by relatives or other persons at the Office of Chief Medical Examiner between February 14 and April 11, 1972. Of these 1000 cases, however, almost two-fifths died of natural causes, particularly cardiovascular disease. When the remaining decedents were grouped according to violent or unnatural cause-of-death categories and were subdivided as alcoholics, narcotics abusers, both, or neither, the number of cases in these subgroups was often too small for detailed analysis. Moreover, there is undoubtedly some seasonal bias in a sample of decedents obtained during a two-month period.

In order to obtain more cases in violent or unnatural cause-of-death categories, with a minimum amount of temporal bias, the sample for the main study described in these pages consists of almost twice as many adults (1954) who were thought to have died unnaturally when initially seen at the Medical Examiner's Office and who were identified by informants during the one-year period from August 20, 1974 to August 19, 1975. It was subsequently determined that nearly all died as a result of homicide, suicide, accident, alcoholism, narcotism, or acute drug poisoning. As in the pilot study, the sample was limited to adults, mainly because of the very small proportion of younger decedents who exhibit postmortem physical evidence of alcoholism (2) and the greater ease of comparison with national or large-scale community drinking practice surveys (3).

A small number of decedents who would have been eligible for the main study but who were either identified by fingerprints, dental records, or in some other manner than by an informant, and those who remained unidentified by the police, were excluded from the sample. There are about 100 unidentified adult decedents in New York City each year. Those decedents who were identified when neither of the staff interviewers was present were also excluded.

A relatively small number of persons whose deaths were certified as being due to natural causes, but who were otherwise identified as alcoholics or narcotics abusers remain in the sample; almost all of them were alcoholics. Likewise, a few victims with no evidence of alcohol or narcotics-related problems whose deaths were initially thought to be unnatural—but were subsequently certified as having natural causes—have been left in the sample. These decedents were all reported to be heavy drinkers, but without any related problems. Heavy drinking without any evidence of related problems was not a criterion for classifying decedents as alcoholics although many were classified as such on the basis of physical evidence.

Informant Questionnaire

The primary data sources in the study were a questionnaire given to informants when they identified decedents at the Medical Examiner's Office (Appendix A) and a postmortem physical findings form (Appendix B). Background data are routinely obtained from informants when they identify decedents at the Office of Chief Medical Examiner and are recorded on an "Identification of Body Form." These data are: relationship of informant to decedent; last time decedent was seen or heard by informant; decedent's age, sex, color, marital status, occupation, and residence. The place and date of

2010-50M-806082(77) ⬤ 346

OFFICE OF CHIEF MEDICAL EXAMINER
OF THE CITY OF NEW YORK

IDENTIFICATION OF BODY

STATE OF NEW YORK
CITY AND COUNTY OF NEW YORK, ss.:
BOROUGH OF

....age.................., residing at

....in the ....

being duly sworn, deposes and says: That   he is a..

of the person whose body was found at.., 19 .....,

and subsequently sent to the Office of Chief Medical Examiner; that deponent has seen the................................

of said deceased, and has every reason to believe that the body now recorded at the Office of Chief Medical

Examiner as..

is...who was last seen or heard from by deponent on

...., 19 ....

    Deponent therefore prays that   identification of said deceased person be accepted by the Chief

Medical Examiner of The City of New York.

Age:......................... Sex:.......................... Color:..........................

Marital Status: ....

Occupation: ....

Residence: ....

Sworn to before me this

   day of.............................19 ......   X...

Identified to:..Death Ctf. issued by:...............................Date:............................

death are also noted on this form. A staff interviewer recorded this information on a study questionnaire and the Medical Examiner's identification form at the same time.

The decedent's place of birth is added to the death certificate by the funeral director and was also obtained for this study. Other characteristics of the dead person recorded in our study were religion, education, and length of residence in New York City, as well as causes of death and drinking or drug problems of immediate family members. Men's service in the U.S. Armed Forces was elicited; this question was added to the interview on September 5, 1974, after 5 percent of the cases were done.

Informant Classification of Alcoholics and Narcotics Abusers

For the purposes of this study, it was necessary to devise questions that would allow informants to identify decedents as alcoholics or drug abusers simply, and without feeling threatened themselves. Most of the earliest epidemiological surveys of alcoholism have relied chiefly on questions about difficulties in life functioning due to drinking (4) that are based on Keller's definition of alcoholism: "a chronic disease manifested by repeated implicative drinking so as to cause injury to the drinker's health or to his social or economic functioning" (5). Irrespective of the screening questions used, the major issue in attempting to identify alcoholics, alive or deceased, in surveys is the considerable underreporting due to conscious or unconscious denial by self-respondents or informants.

Apart from denial of alcoholism, questions about health, family, job, or money problems due to drinking are subject to variation in defining what constitutes a "problem" depending on the informant's sociocultural group. Some alcoholics, for example, are labeled by relatives as "heavy drinkers only" without any resulting problems despite contrary evidence. Most of those reported in our study to be "heavy drinkers only" were likely to have had unreported problems because of too much drinking. By the same token, informants' reports also produce some false positives, including persons whose drinking problems are temporary responses to crises and some whose problems are minimally related to drinking. Still others, perhaps identified by zealous prohibitionists, are light or moderate drinkers even by stringent quantity–frequency indices. Nonetheless, questions about troubles due to drinking, in addition to being nonthreatening and simple, are a more accurate means of identifying known alcoholics than are quantity–frequency indices or attitudinal and behavioral alcohol scales (6).

It should be noted, parenthetically, that informants or "proxy" respondents have proved as likely (7) or more likely (6) than self-respondents to report troubles due to drinking for previously identified alcoholics. The relatives or other persons identifying decedents at the Medical Examiner's Office are, of course, all "proxy" respondents.

In contrast to alcohol consumption, any use of illicit drugs, such as heroin, is generally considered to be a problem regardless of the quantity used. Narcotics are more likely than alcohol to seriously involve the user with the criminal justice system. Heroin is certainly less socially acceptable and carries more of a stigma than alcohol does. Since narcotics use alone would be considered a problem in most sociocultural groups, the question on drug use in our study is nonspecific rather than being addressed to specific problems in life functioning related to drug abuse.

Informants who are not closely related to decedents or have not seen them for a long time may not know about any problems due to drinking or drug use. Informants may also deny such problems because of the stigma attached to alcoholism and narcotism or because they rightly or wrongly believe that an admission of drinking or drug problems may jeopardize life- or health-insurance payments. In contrast to most other studies of alcoholism or other drug problems which do not include a criterion measure, the informants' responses in our study can be validated by physical evidence of alcoholism or narcotism.

The questioning of persons identifying decedents about alcoholism or problem drinking and other drug use is completely within the routine course of the official investigation by the Chief Medical Examiner's Office into the circumstances of death and the prior medical history. Such questions, however, are not usually worded in the same way for all informants; various medical examiner office workers ask about alcohol and other drug use differently. For the purposes of this study, the questions about drinking and drug problems were always asked in an identical manner.

Did the decedent *ever* have any health problems because of drinking (alcoholic beverages)?
Did the decedent *ever* have any family, money, job, or other problems because of drinking?
Did the decedent *ever* have any problems because of drug use?
IF YES: What drug(s) did the decedent take?

"Heavy drinking only" without related problems was not sufficient to classify decedents as informant-classified alcoholics. Unfortunately, informants were not asked about the quantity or frequency of alcoholic beverages which decedents usually drank so that "heavy drinking only" was a volunteered response. If all informants had been asked identical questions about alcohol consumption, decedents might have been classified as alcoholics on the basis of very heavy drinking alone despite a denial of related problems. On the other hand, decedents were classified as alcoholics or drug abusers if their principal activity — what they were doing most of the past year — was reported to be drinking or drug-taking.

If any problems due to drinking were mentioned by informants, questions were asked about the last time such problems occurred, where the decedents had sought help, and the last time they received any help. When problems due to drug use were reported, informants were similarly asked about the last time any problems had occurred. When use of heroin, morphine, or methadone was reported, informants were queried about the decedents' participation in a methadone maintenance treatment program (MMTP) in order to evaluate the presence or absence of methadone in toxicologic tests. In addition, informants were asked if the decedent had ever been hospitalized for liver trouble and, if so, when. In the responses to this question, hepatitis, probably related to narcotics use, was distinguished from other liver trouble probably related to alcoholism.

The last two questions asked of informants dealt with causes of death and drinking or drug problems in the decedent's immediate family. Members of the immediate family were defined as parents, siblings, spouse, and children. These two series of questions were included to ascertain familial patterns in alcoholism and narcotism in conjunction with violent death.

Physical Classification of Alcoholics and Narcotics Abusers

The date and place of death from the Medical Examiner's "Identification of Body Form" (p. 15) were recorded on the physical findings form used in this study. Other postmortem data recorded on this study form were: evidence of drinking at the scene; cause-of-death certification; type of examination; autopsy findings; blood or brain alcohol concentration (BAC); and toxicologic findings of other drug ingestion just prior to death. When narcotism was noted on the back of the death certificate, it was also written on the study form. Evidence of narcotics use may be difficult to discern in the written autopsy report, so narcotism is occasionally written on the back of the certificate, when it does not contribute to the cause of death.

Physical classification of decedents as alcoholics, for purposes of the study, was made on the basis of either cause-of-death certification or on autopsy findings and prior medical history. The relevant death certificate categories are: acute alcoholism, chronic alcoholism, both conditions, and alcoholism in conjunction with another cause of death, whether it is natural, accidental, narcotism, or acute mixed-drug poisoning. Death from acute alcoholism is defined as being caused by recent drinking usually, but not necessarily, associated with elevated BACs of 0.30 percent or above (1). Alcohol may not be present, however, in the tissues of persons who were hospitalized or were comatose for more than a day before death. Death from chronic alcoholism is caused by long medical complications resulting from periods of excessive alcohol use. Death from acute and chronic alcoholism refers to recent heavy drinking together with long periods of alcoholism. At least fifteen years' steady drinking usually precedes a diagnosis of liver damage, so that cirrhosis rarely occurs in alcoholics younger than 35 years of age (8). Consequently, some younger decedents in our sample would not yet have had physical evidence of their excessive drinking, and may have been misclassified as nonalcoholics in the absence of any problems related to drinking, as reported by the informants.

It should be noted here that the overall reported mortality from alcohol-related disorders (not only in our medical examiner cases) is seriously understated because of a reluctance to certify alcoholism as the cause of death when it is possible to assign another cause or complication (9). Thus alcohol is frequently not mentioned even though it is a contributing factor in accidental deaths or in deaths resulting from a combination of alcohol and other drugs. Furthermore, in New York City well over nine-tenths of the mortality from cirrhosis of the liver can be attributed to alcohol, yet less than one-half of such deaths are recorded as liver cirrhosis associated with alcoholism (10). Most are recorded as cirrhosis without mention of alcoholism, despite the very high incidence of alcoholism as an etiological factor in cirrhosis of the liver described in postmortem and clinical studies (11). "Fears of stigmatization by the certifying physician and the nature of the death certificate itself," which has no provision to indicate predisposing alcoholism, along with legal ramifications, are the most important factors in this considerable underreporting (10).

Most of the mortality statistics have been based on the single diagnostic entry selected as the underlying cause of death. Even when a contributory cause such as alcoholism or intemperate drinking has been listed, very few studies have utilized multiple cause-of-death data (12). This selective underreporting of alcoholism as the underlying or contributing cause of death may significantly affect the recorded variation among racial and socioeconomic groups in such mortality statistics (9).

The postmortem findings from complete or partial autopsies each of which could be attributed to alcoholism in this medical examiner population nine of ten times are: moderate or severe fatty change in the liver, cirrhosis of the liver, and, rarely, pancreatitis, or ruptured esophageal varices (if these findings were unrelated to some other disease or condition). Partial autopsies, which may only encompass an abdominal incision, are done in a small proportion of cases usually to confirm a suspicion of alcoholism by inspection of the liver.

Physical classification of decedents as narcotics abusers was made either on the basis of cause-of-death certification, toxicologic findings of morphine, which is the metabolite of heroin, or methadone, or "back-of-certificate narcotism." Heroin, it should be noted, is metabolized rapidly to morphine in the body so that morphine would be detected in toxicologic tests following recent heroin use (13). If narcotics use was implicated elsewhere, toxicologic findings of quinine or lidocaine alone were also considered criteria for recent use. Quinine and, more recently, lidocaine are common adulterants of heroin in New York City and may remain in the body longer than heroin. Since quinine is an ingredient in tonic water and some medicines, such use of the latter had to be excluded in order to consider quinine alone evidence of heroin use. Lidocaine was considered evidence of recent heroin use only if death did not occur in a hospital, since it is possible to administer lidocaine medically.

The relevant death certificate categories are "acute and/or chronic narcotism" alone or in conjunction with another cause of death. Acute narcotism is based on finding a fresh intravenous injection site and very enlarged and heavy lungs (14). Chronic narcotism is based on finding "perivenous" scarring or "track marks" or subcutaneous injection scars.

Barbiturates and tranquilizers were the two non-narcotic drugs most often found in toxicologic tests on alcoholics, narcotics abusers, and nonabusers. They were often present in suicide victims, most of whom were neither alcoholics nor narcotics abusers. Barbiturates were also the substance most likely to be found in the few cases of acute (non-narcotic) drug poisoning in our study. In addition, Darvon (propoxyphene) and carbon monoxide were sometimes detected by toxicologic tests. Carbon monoxide was most often associated with fires.

Sample Composition

The sample was designed to include as many identified decedents eighteen years of age or older as possible (in a one-year period) whose death was caused by homicide, suicide, accident, alcohol, or other drugs. The interviewing of informants at the Medical Examiner's Office was conducted on Saturdays and Sundays, as well as on weekdays, for the twelve-month period beginning August 20, 1974. A seven-day-per-week work schedule over a full year was utilized in order to avoid any systematic daily, monthly, or seasonal bias. This extensive data collection was also necessary to obtain sufficient cases for detailed subgroup analyses.

The study sample of 1954 Medical Examiner cases, consequently, comprises 3 to 4 percent of all adults who died in four of the five City boroughs (excluding Brooklyn) and about one-half of all the violent deaths of adults investigated by the Chief Medical Examiner's Office during that twelve-month period (15). The sample included about one-half of all adult homicide, motor vehicle accident, and drug-dependence victims; a somewhat larger percentage of all suicides; and a smaller percentage of those who died from other accidents.

According to the New York City Department of Health Vital Statistics for 1974, approximately 54,000 adults died in the Bronx, Manhattan, Queens, and Staten Island; 65 percent were at least 65 years old, 54 percent were men, and 83 percent were white (15). In contrast, the study decedents, as shown in Table 2.1 are much younger, predominantly male, and more often nonwhite. Specifically, 65 percent of these sample cases were less than 45 years old, 76 percent were men, and 60 percent were white. In the 1970 census, adults who resided in one of these four boroughs were somewhat older than the sample, more often women, and 81 percent white (16). New York City mortality statistics for 1974 and U.S. census population data for 1970 are the most recent compilations available for comparative purposes.

Parenthetically, mortality rates by race in the New York City vital statistics for 1974 do not include a separate category for Puerto Ricans, who are classified as white in 91 percent of the cases and nonwhite in 9 percent, according to the Community Council of Greater New York. For comparability in Table 2.1, study decedents of Hispanic descent who comprise 21 percent of the sample are also classified as white or nonwhite in these same proportions.

Puerto Ricans are overrepresented among medical examiner cases. About 16 percent of our sample were either born in Puerto Rico or had at least one Puerto Rican parent, whereas only about one-half that percentage of Puerto Rican adults defined in this manner (8%) lived in the study area in 1970 (16). It may be assumed that the 1974 City mortality statistics include a smaller proportion of Puerto Ricans than the sample does.

A disproportionately large number of study decedents resided in Manhattan compared to the relative proportions for overall mortality

Table 2–1. Demographic Comparisons: Our Study, New York City Mortality, and Population Statistics (persons eighteen years of age or older)

	STUDY DECEDENTS, 1974–75 ($N = 1954$)	N.Y.C. MORTALITY, 1974[a] ($N = 54,000$)	N.Y.C. POPULATION, 1970[b] ($N = 3,900,000$)
Sex			
Male	76.2%	53.9%	45.4%
Female	23.8	46.1	54.6
Total	100%	100%	100%
Age			
18–24	18.3%	2.0%[c]	15.3%
25–44	46.5	7.2	35.3
45–64	25.0	25.8	32.4
65 or older	10.2	65.0	17.0
Total	100%	100%	100%
Color			
White	60.2%[d]	83.3%	80.8%
Nonwhite	39.8	16.7	19.2
Total	100%	100%	100%
Residence			
Bronx	24.7%	30.4%	26.0%
Manhattan	46.4	23.6	31.2
Queens	16.5	33.8	37.8
Staten Island	1.6	4.6	5.0
Other[e]	10.2	6.5	n.a.*
Unknown	0.6	1.1	n.a.
Total	100%	100%	100%

a. *Source:* New York City Department of Health, Bureau of Health, Statistics and Analysis, *Vital Statistics, 1974.* (Brooklyn residents excluded.) (15)

b. *Source:* U.S. Bureau of the Census, 1970 Decennial Census data obtained from Community Council of Greater New York. (Brooklyn residents excluded.) (16)

c. Percent 18–24 estimated since age group is 15–24.

d. Puerto Ricans and other Latin Americans in study are distributed 91% white and 9% nonwhite as recommended by Community Council of Greater New York to make study data comparable to government statistics.

e. Includes Brooklyn residents.

*n.a.: not applicable.

and population in Manhattan (Table 2.1) (15, 16). Forty-six percent of the sample and less than one-third of the comparison groups were Manhattan residents. Likewise, 55 percent of the sample died in Manhattan. A correspondingly smaller proportion of the sample were Queens residents at the time of death. The relatively large number of decedents in the sample whose last residence and place of death was in Manhattan probably reflects both the larger proportion of Manhattan cases brought to the Medical Examiner's Office, as previously mentioned, and also the greater incidence of violent deaths there.

The study cases as well as this Medical Examiner population in general may be characterized as predominantly black or Hispanic men, less than 45 years of age, who lived and died in Manhattan. The sample comprised roughly one-half of all violent deaths of adults investigated by the New York City Medical Examiner's Office, and is representative of the total Medical Examiner population during the study year in the same age and cause-of-death categories.

References

1. P. W. Haberman and M. M. Baden, "Alcoholism and Violent Death," *Quarterly Journal of Studies on Alcohol 35*: 1974, pp. 221–31.
2. P. Sundby, *Alcoholism and Mortality*, New Brunswick, N. J.: Rutgers Center of Alcohol Studies, 1967, pp. 189 and 206.
3. See for example D. Cahalan, *Problem Drinkers*, San Francisco: Jossey-Bass, 1970; H. A. Mulford, "Drinking and Deviant Drinking, U.S.A., 1963," *Quarterly Journal of Studies on Alcohol 25*: 1964, pp. 634–50; M. B. Bailey, P. W. Haberman, and H. Alksne, "The Epidemiology of Alcoholism in an Urban Residential Area," *Quarterly Journal of Studies on Alcohol 26*: 1965, pp. 19–40; and P. W. Haberman and J. Sheinberg, "Implicative Drinking Reported in a Household Survey," *Quarterly Journal of Studies on Alcohol 28*: 1967, pp. 538–43.
4. For example, M. B. Bailey, P. W. Haberman, and H. Alksne; and P. W. Haberman and J. Sheinberg. See ref. 3 above.
5. M. Keller, "Definition of Alcoholism," *Quarterly Journal of Studies on Alcohol 21*: 1960, pp. 125–34.
6. H. A. Mulford and R. W. Wilson, *Identifying Problem Drinkers in a Household Health Survey*. Washington, D.C.: Public Health Service Publication No. 1000, Series 2, No. 16, 1966.
7. M. B. Bailey, P. W. Haberman, and J. Sheinberg, "Identifying Alcoholics in Population Surveys: A Report on Reliability," *Quarterly Journal of Studies on Alcohol 27*: 1966, pp. 300–15.
8. S. Sherlock, *Diseases of the Liver and Biliary System*, Philadelphia: F. A. Davis, 4th ed., 1968, pp. 412–25.
9. Metropolitan Life Insurance Co. "Alcoholism: A Growing Medical-Social Problem," *Statistical Bulletin 48*: April, 1967, pp. 7–10.

10. M. M. Baden, "Alcoholism as Related to Drug Addiction: A Medical Examiner's View," in *Drug Abuse: Current Concepts and and Research*, W. Keup, ed., Springfield, Ill.: Charles C. Thomas, 1972.

11. See for example: ref. 8 above; A. J. Patek, Chap. 18, in *Diseases of the Liver*, L. Schiff, ed., Philadelphia: J. B. Lippincott, 3rd ed., 1969, pp. 676–80; E. Rubin, "The Spectrum of Alcoholic Liver Injury," in *The Liver*, E. A. Gall and F. K. Mostofi, eds., Baltimore: Williams and Wilkins, 1973, pp. 199–217.

12. P. W. Haberman, "The Reliability and Validity of the Data," in *Poverty and Health: A Sociological Analysis*, J. Kosa, A. Antonovsky, and I. K. Zola, eds., Cambridge, Mass.: Harvard University Press, 1969, pp. 343–83.

13. M. M. Baden, "Investigation of Deaths from Drug Abuse," in: *Mediolegal Investigation of Death: Guidelines for the Application of Pathology to Criminal Investigation*, W. U. Spitz and R. S. Fisher, eds., Springfield, Ill.: Charles C. Thomas, 1973, pp. 485–508.

14. C. Cherubin et al., "The Epidemiology of Death in Narcotic Addicts," *American Journal of Epidemiology 96:* 1972, pp. 11–22.

15. *Vital Statistics by Health Areas and Health Center Districts, 1974.* New York City Department of Health, Bureau of Health Statistics and Analysis, 1976.

16. 1970 Decennial Census Data, U.S. Department of Commerce, Bureau of the Census, from the Community Council of Greater New York, Department of Research and Program Planning Information.

3

Classifying Decedents as Alcoholics and Narcotics Abusers

The various methods used to identify alcoholics and narcotics abusers in the sample are presented in this chapter. Informant and physical criteria for classification of decedents as substance abusers were described in Chapter 2. Overall, 58 percent of the 1954 cases in the sample had an identified problem with alcohol and/or narcotics. Two-fifths were classified as alcoholics and almost three-tenths as narcotics abusers, including more than one-tenth classified as both. The sample proportions are: alcoholics 29.7 percent, narcotics abusers 17.3 percent, both conditions 11.4 percent, and neither condition 41.6 percent.

The proportions of alcoholics and narcotics abusers classified by specific methods are summarized in Table 3.1. Fifty-six percent of the alcoholics and 71 percent of the narcotics abusers were classified as such by informants, with or without corroborating physical evidence. Alcoholics classified by informants included 39 percent who were also classified by physical evidence and 17 percent who were not. For the narcotics abusers, the comparable proportions are 51 percent and 20 percent, respectively. Even larger proportions—83 percent of the alcoholics and 80 percent of the narcotics abusers— were so classified on the basis of physical evidence, with or without informant affirmation.

Postmortem medical procedures to test for alcoholism or narcotics

Table 3–1. Method of Classification of Decedents as Alcoholics and Narcotics Abusers

METHOD OF CLASSIFICATION	N:	ALCOHOLICS[a] (803)	NARCOTICS ABUSERS[a] (561)
Informant only			
No autopsy or toxicologic tests[b]		6.5%	7.0%
Autopsy (alcoholism) or toxicologic tests (narcotics abusers)[c]		10.6 (17.1)	13.0 (20.0)
Physical evidence only			
Cause-of-death certification		18.1	19.3
Autopsy[d] or toxicologic findings[e]		26.4 (44.5)	9.8[f] (29.1)
Both informant and physical evidence			
Cause-of-death certification		28.0	35.5
Autopsy[d] or toxicologic findings[e]		10.5 (38.5)	15.5 (51.0)
Total		100%	100%

a. Those who were both alcoholics and narcotics abusers ($N = 222$) included in both groups.

b. External examination, including ten with autopsy but examination of liver not possible.

c. Includes two with external examination and possible evidence of alcoholism.

d. Autopsy findings for classification as alcoholic: moderate or severe (bright yellow) fatty change in liver, cirrhosis of liver, pancreatitis, or ruptured esophageal varices, not attributable to other disease or condition.

e. Toxicologic findings for classification as narcotics abuser: morphine (heroin metabolite) and methadone.

f. Includes nine with only "back-of-certificate" narcotism.

use cannot always provide conclusive results. Because of coma, severe damage to the body, or a long enough interval between death and postmortem physical examination for the body to become decomposed, an autopsy inspection of the liver for evidence of chronic alcoholism may not be revealing. Similarly, toxicologic tests for recent drug ingestion may be of no value if the person dies in a hospital after a sufficient interval to permit metabolism of suspected drugs. For a small proportion of decedents who were classified as alcoholics or narcotics abusers by informants only (7% in each case), the study criteria could not be met because autopsies for evidence of alcoholism or toxicologic tests for evidence of recent use of narcotics were not performed. Likewise, criterion postmortem medical procedures were not performed on a few persons whose cause of death was certified as alcoholism and/or narcotism (10% in all subgroups).

With regard to physical evidence in our study, both alcoholics and narcotics abusers were classified as such by cause of death (based on both medical history and physical findings) more often than by autopsy or toxicologic findings of substance abuse with some other cause of death (Table 3.1). More than twice as many decedents were classified as narcotics abusers on the basis of cause-of-death certification (55%) than on toxicologic findings of morphine (the heroin metabolite) or methadone alone (24%).

Although the difference was less marked with alcoholics, cause-of-death certification (46%) was more often the method of classification than autopsy findings, such as liver damage due to alcohol (37%). These study results, it should be noted, are remarkably similar to those obtained about three years earlier in the pilot study (1).

Corroborating Evidence of Substance Abuse

Of those persons who died of alcoholism, 88 percent had autopsy evidence of chronic physical problems due to this condition, and the remainder died of acute alcoholism with or without some other concomitant cause, as shown in Table 3.2. Similarly, for 86 percent of those who died of narcotism, there was toxicologic evidence of morphine or methadone. This would indicate recent use which elicited an acute reaction to the narcotic, an adulterant, or concomitant drug and alcohol use (2).

Additional confirmation by informants of health problems related to alcohol or narcotics use was obtained through a history of hospitalization for hepatitis or other liver trouble. All but four of the 119 decedents (97%) who were reported to be hospitalized for liver trouble other than hepatitis were classified as alcoholics by informant and/or by physical criteria, and 80 percent of the 80 decedents with a reported hospitalization for hepatitis — most likely the result of using unsterile syringes — were classified as narcotics abusers. Similarly, 53 percent of the 239 decedents reported to be heavy drinkers without

Table 3–2. Postmortem Physical Findings When Cause of Death was Alcoholism and/or Narcotism

| PHYSICAL FINDINGS | CAUSE OF DEATH[a] | |
| | Alcoholism | Narcotism |
N:	(370)	(307)
Autopsy evidence of chronic alcoholism	(90.0%)[b]	(91.9%)[b]
No	12.0%[c]	72.7%
Yes	88.0	27.3
Total	100%	100%
BAC	(43.4%)[b]	(87.3%)[b]
Negative	33.1%	67.5%
.01 – .09%	25.6	18.3
.10 – .29%	31.3	13.8
.30% or above	10.0	0.3
Total	100%	100%
Other toxicology	(43.2%)[b]	(88.6%)[b]
Negative or no mood-altering drugs	52.5%	8.1%
Narcotics[d]	26.3	86.4
Other mood-altering drugs[e]	21.3	5.5
Total	100%	100%

a. Cause of death both alcoholism and narcotism ($N = 60$) included in both groups.

b. Percentages in parentheses are proportions with autopsy performed and BAC or other toxicology obtained.

c. Cause of death was certified as acute alcoholism with or without other cause, i.e., natural condition, accident, or mixed drug poisoning.

d. Irrespective of absence or presence of other mood-altering drugs.

e. Primarily (79.2%) barbiturates and/or tranquilizers.

any related problems were classified as alcoholics by physical evidence confirming the likelihood of unreported problems due to excessive drinking. An additional 20 percent were narcotics abusers without any evidence of alcoholism confirmed in this study.

Decedents reported to be "heavy drinkers only" were somewhat more likely to have a positive blood or brain alcohol concentration (BAC) than those classified by informants as alcoholics (see Table 3.3, p. 31). Sixty-five percent of the "heavy drinkers" and 58 percent of the alcoholics classified by informants had a positive BAC and, more significantly, over two-fifths in each subgroup (44.6% heavy drinkers, 42.1% informant-classified alcoholics) had BACs of 0.10 percent or above, indicating legal impairment or intoxication from alcohol for driving motor vehicles (3). In contrast, only 33 percent of the decedents without any problems related to drinking or heavy drinking reported by informants had a positive BAC and just 18 percent had alcohol levels of 0.10 percent or above.

The absence of strong sanctions against alcoholism may contribute to the admission of "heavy drinking" alone, when acknowledgment of related problems would be more accurate (4). Some social problems are more prevalent among poor people and minority groups, irrespective of drinking patterns. In such cases the association between economic or family problems and excessive drinking may be obscured, resulting in fewer reported problems related to drinking (4). The reasons for much of the denial of problems related to "heavy drinking" in our study may be due to these same factors, i.e., the lack of strong sanctions against alcoholism and low socioeconomic status.

Health problems due to drinking were reported more than twice as often as was any other kind of difficulty — by 67 percent of the 446 informants reporting one or more problem. In large-scale epidemiological surveys, however, family, money, or job problems have been mentioned more often than they were in our study (5), which probably reflects the difference between studies of live and dead persons. However, all but one alcoholic and one narcotics abuser among the decedents whose principal activity during the past year was reported to be drinking or taking drugs were also identified as having had problems related to substance abuse. Well over half of these 95 cases died of alcoholism (70.0% of 43) or narcotism (57.7% of 52).

Acute versus Chronic Substance Abuse

The physical evidence used in our study to classify decedents as alcoholics — mainly autopsy findings of liver damage — is a manifestation of chronic alcoholism. On the other hand, toxicologic findings of morphine or methadone used to classify decedents as narcotics abusers indicate recent use of narcotics and probably acute reaction to those narcotics. Thus medical examiner evidence of acute alcoholism and chronic narcotism was obtained primarily from the cause-of-death certification.

Of the 370 persons whose cause of death included alcoholism, 63 percent were certified as chronic, 20 percent as acute and chronic and the remainder, 17 percent, acute only or alcoholism unspecified. As indicated in Table 3.3 however, the BAC was not measured in most of these cases (56.8%) because too much time had elapsed between the last drink and death, or because the evidence of chronic alcoholism seemed sufficient to consider it the cause of death. Forty-one percent of the persons who died of alcoholism and 14 percent of those who died of narcotism had a BAC of 0.10 percent or higher. The BAC for 13 percent of those who died of alcoholism was 0.30 percent or above, which indicates that death from acute alcoholism was possible. Moreover, alcohol is metabolized by the body at a rate of approximately 0.015 percent per hour (6), so that a larger proportion of the decedents undoubtedly had peak concentrations of 0.30 percent or higher at some time shortly before death.

Some persons whose deaths are due to acute alcoholism may have been nonabusers with no previous problems related to their drinking. However, other evidence of alcoholism in our study such as related problems reported by informants or autopsy findings of liver damage due to excessive drinking was present in eight of the ten cases who died of acute alcoholism without any other cause of death. Thus death from acute alcoholism seems to occur rarely after a solitary drinking episode by previous nonabusers.

There are still other factors which complicate the interpretation of BAC results in living as well as dead persons. First of all, effects of the same concentration of alcohol vary among individuals, and even in the same individual at different times. Second, the amount of alcohol consumption needed to attain a specific BAC varies directly with a person's body weight. Finally, nonabusers by all other criteria may

Table 3-3. BAC According to Informant Classification of Alcoholics

	N:	INFORMANT CLASSIFICATION		
BAC		Alcoholics (233)[a]	Heavy Drinkers Only (175)[a]	Nonalcoholics (1018)[a]
Negative		42.1%	35.4%	67.3%
.01 – .09%		15.9	20.0	15.1
.10% or above		42.1	44.6	17.6
Total		100%	100%	100%

a. Total numbers and proportions with BAC obtained are: alcoholics 446 and 52.2%; heavy drinkers only 239 and 73.2%; nonalcoholics 1269 and 80.2%.

on a given occasion have an elevated BAC so that alcohol contributed to their deaths even though they were not alcoholics. The usual effects of different quantities of alcohol consumption are described in Table 3.4 (7).

Narcotics addiction itself causes virtually no organ damage (8); external scars, commonly referred to as "track marks" are the most frequent indication of chronic heroin use (9). Evidence of chronic narcotism was usually found on the cause-of-death certification. Chronic (without acute) narcotism was most likely to be the cause of death in conjunction with infections associated with narcotics use, or such a relationship could be inferred when narcotism was noted on the back of the certificate without any evidence of recent use. As previously noted, morphine or methadone was found in almost nine-tenths of the toxicologic tests on persons who died of narcotism, indicating that a fatal acute reaction probably had occurred. Thus when narcotism was listed as the cause of death, it was most often certified as acute or acute and chronic (intravenous) narcotism.

Admission of Problems by Informants

The relationship and proximity of informants and decedents may provide some explanation for patterns of admission or denial of decedents' drinking or drug problems. In Table 3.5, alcoholics and narcotics abusers are subdivided according to the means used for their classification—by informant or by physical evidence only. Within the subgroups classified as alcoholics and narcotics abusers, there are no major differences according to informant—decedent relationship. Thus no particular relative—spouse, child, parent, or sibling—seemed to be more or less likely to acknowledge the decedents' alcoholism or narcotism. Between the two substances, however, there are marked differences in the relationship between informants and decedents. Siblings or parents each accounted for about one-third (32.0% and 32.4%) of the informants for narcotics abusers, while siblings (28.9%) were the most frequent informants for alcoholics, making identifications more than twice as often as did parents (13.9%).

Table 3–4. Effects of Alcohol Consumption (adapted from Cross, ref. 7)

QUANTITY CONSUMED IN ONE HOUR BY PERSONS WEIGHING ABOUT 150 POUNDS[a]	APPROXIMATE BAC	PROBABLE EFFECTS[b]	TIME NECESSARY FOR COMPLETE METABOLISM
1 highball or cocktail ($1\frac{1}{2}$ oz. whiskey) or $5\frac{1}{2}$ oz. ordinary wine or 2 bottles beer (24 oz.)[c]	0.03%	No noticeable effects on behavior	2 hours
3 highballs or cocktails ($4\frac{1}{2}$ oz.) or $16\frac{1}{2}$ oz. (1 pint) ordinary wine or 6 bottles beer (72 oz.)	0.09%	Emotional instability, decrease in fine skills, some mental confusion, drowsiness, decreased inhibitions, loss of critical judgement	6 hours
5 highballs or cocktails ($7\frac{1}{2}$ oz.) or $27\frac{1}{2}$ oz. (1.6 pints) ordinary wine or 10 bottles beer (120 oz.)	0.15%	Confusion, impairment of fine coordination, intoxication, abnormalities of gross bodily functions and mental faculties	10 hours
10 highballs or cocktails (15 oz.) or 55 oz. (3.2. pints) ordinary wine or more	0.30% or higher	Incoordination, apathy, general inertia, decreased response to stimuli, impaired consciousness, sleep or stupor, coma, death	20 hours

a. For persons weighing considerably more or less than 150 pounds, quantities consumed to attain BAC, probable effects, and time taken for alcohol to leave body will be correspondingly more or less.

b. Possible effects will diminish as BAC diminishes. Effects for specific BACs vary among individuals and in same individual at different times. Absorption of alcohol is delayed in presence of food, thus diminishing peak effects and is accelerated in drinks mixed with plain or carbonated water, thus increasing peak effects.

c. Approximately this quantity every 2 hours is necessary to maintain BAC roughly constant.

Table 3-5. Relationship and Proximity of Informants and Decedents According to Method of Classification as Alcoholics and Narcotics Abusers

METHOD OF CLASSIFICATION: N:	ALCOHOLICS[a]			NARCOTICS ABUSERS[a]		
	Total Identified (803)	Informant[b] (446)	Physical Evidence Only[c] (357)	Total Identified (561)	Informant[b] (398)	Physical Evidence Only[c] (163)
Informant-decedent relationship						
Spouse	14.7%	15.9%	13.2%	11.8%	12.1%	11.0%
Son, daughter	12.0	12.3	11.8	3.2	2.5	4.9
Father, mother	13.9	12.8	15.4	32.4	32.9	31.3
Brother, sister	28.9	30.7	26.6	32.0	33.2	29.4
Other relative	17.6	16.4	19.0	13.9	12.3	17.8
Friend	11.1	10.1	12.3	6.2	6.5	5.5
Other	1.7	1.8	1.7	0.4	0.5	–
Total	100%	100%	100%	100%	100%	100%
When informant last spoke to decedent						
Within one day of death	33.9%	28.3%	40.9%	35.7%	37.4%	31.3%
Within one week	28.4	29.1	27.5	31.4	30.9	32.5
Within one month	20.8	24.2	16.5	20.1	20.1	20.2
More than one month	16.9	18.4	15.1	12.9	11.6	16.0
Total	100%	100%	100%	100%	100%	100%
Lived in same household[d]						
Yes	22.5%	20.6%	24.9%	30.1%	32.9%	23.3%
No	77.5	79.4	75.1	69.9	67.1	76.7
Total	100%	100%	100%	100%	100%	100%

a. Those who were both alcoholics and narcotics abusers (N = 222) included in both groups.
b. Informant admission, with or without physical evidence of condition.
c. Informant denial of condition.
d. Only asked of informants who last spoke to decedent within one month prior to death or more recently. Informants who last spoke to decedent more than one month prior to death were assumed not to live in same household as decedent.

Children were much more likely to be informants for alcoholics, and parents were more often informants for narcotics abusers, irrespective of admission or denial of related problems. These informant variations primarily reflect the considerable age difference at the time of death between the alcoholics and narcotics abusers; 54 percent of the alcoholics were 40 years of age or older, whereas 60 percent of the narcotics abusers were less than 30 years old.

The closeness or proximity of informants and decedents indicates that there are differences in admission or denial of alcohol and narcotics problems (Table 3.5). Alcoholics who last spoke to the informants within one day of their death were more often classified as such by physical evidence only (40.9%) rather than by informants (28.3%). Narcotics abusers with the same proximity to the informants were more often classified as such by them (37.4%) than by physical evidence alone (31.3%).

Estimating the proximity between informants and decedents according to whether or not they live in the same household produced comparable results regarding the admission or denial of drug problems. Alcoholics living with informants were more likely to be identified by physical evidence alone than by informants, and the order was reversed for narcotics abusers. However, 74 percent of the 483 decedents who had been living with informants, but only 25 percent of the 1471 who had not been living with informants, spoke to decedents within one day of their death, which leads us to conclude that these findings are not independent of those described in the preceding paragraph.

Therefore, relatives and friends in close proximity to alcoholics were more likely to deny any drinking problems than those with less recent contact. In contrast, relatives and friends in close proximity to narcotics abusers were more likely to acknowledge problems due to narcotics use than those with less recent contact. The reasons for these differences are unclear. However, the legality of alcoholic beverages, the relatively slow progression of alcoholism symptoms, and the tolerance or presence of heavy social drinking or incipient problem drinking in the alcoholic's family may effectively make the informant less aware of the condition. Narcotics, in contrast, are illegal and are rapidly addictive substances with legal, economic, and social consequences that are more easily recognizable by those in close proximity to the narcotics abuser. In addition, alcoholism and narcotism may be perceived in a very different manner by informants; much less exposure to heroin or methadone than to alcohol is needed for a user to be classified as an abuser by his associates.

Both tolerant and negative attitudes toward alcoholism have been suggested as possible reasons for the denial of problems related to drinking (10). Strong negative attitudes may deter informants from admitting socially unacceptable behavior such as problem drinking unless it becomes too disruptive, as is more likely with narcotics abuse. With tolerant attitudes, a greater degree of stress may be necessary for the consequences of heavy drinking to be labeled as problems. Narcotics abuse is apt to cause highly stressful situations sooner than alcohol abuse.

The differences between informant admission or denial of alcoholism and narcotism are further substantiated by the classification patterns for decedents with both conditions shown in Table 3.6. Of these 222 cases, 78 percent were classified as narcotics abusers by the informants, but only 54 percent were classified as alcoholics by these same informants. Stated another way, 22 percent of these informants denied the decedents' narcotism, while 46 percent denied their alcoholism. These data suggest that for decedents with both conditions, the consequences of their narcotism were more visible to close observers than the consequences of their alcoholism, most likely be-

Table 3–6. Method for Classifying Decedents Who Were Both Alcoholics and Narcotics Abusers (N = 222)

METHOD OF CLASSIFICATION	ALCOHOLICS[a]	NARCOTICS ABUSERS[b]
Informant only	19.4%	24.3%
Physical evidence only	45.9	22.1
Both informant and physical evidence	34.7	53.6
Total	100%	100%

a. Autopsy findings for classification as alcoholic: moderate or severe (bright yellow) fatty change in liver, cirrhosis of liver, pancreatitis, or ruptured esophageal varices, not attributable to other disease or condition (see description in Chapter 2).

b. Toxicologic findings for classification as narcotics abuser: morphine (heroin metabolite) and methadone.

cause of the differences between the two substances. The illegality, cost, and addictive properties of heroin may account for the greater awareness and acknowledgement of problems that result from its use. An alternative explanation which will be explored in the next chapter is that decedents with both conditions were primarily narcotics abusers rather than alcoholics.

Implications

Forty-seven percent of the alcoholics in our study died of alcoholism, almost always with physical evidence of chronic effects such as liver damage, and 55 percent of the narcotics abusers died of narcotism, usually involving an acute reaction. For those with both conditions, either or both of the substances were cited as the cause of death in 72 percent of the cases. Narcotics alone (27.9%) and both substances together (27.0%) were implicated more often than alcohol alone (16.7%). Thus substance abuse itself was by far the major cause of death among cases in our study classified as alcoholics, narcotics abusers, or both, even though alcohol and other drugs have an appreciable role in suicides, homicides, and fatal accidents.

In studies of chronic diseases, re-examination (or follow-up interviews) have been used to increase the number of survey positives. Because of the remittent nature of rheumatoid arthritis, for example, subjects in one study with relevant symptoms, e.g., joint swelling, tenderness, or pain during motion, observed at either of two examinations were classified as having this disease (11). "By making it quite clear that . . . the [chronic] disease process occurs as a continuum of disturbance, not as a have-it or don't-have-it phenomenon," such procedures have contributed to the epidemiology of rheumatoid disorders and chronic disease in general (12). This scheme is particularly applicable when periodicity and variable progression are important characteristics of the disorder under study. Thus, underreporting or underestimation of chronic conditions like alcoholism and narcotism, which have a high degree of social stigma and may be episodic, can be substantially reduced by using more than one method for identifying subjects.

Similarly, there was a considerable amount of underreporting by informants in our study and smaller, but not inconsequential, proportions of cases without physical evidence of problems. Forty-five percent of the alcoholics and 29 percent of the narcotics abusers were classified by physical evidence only, and about one-fifth in each subgroup (17% alcoholics, 20% narcotics abusers) were classified by informants only. Thus, a sizeable minority of our cases would not have been classified as alcoholics or narcotics abusers if only one procedure had been used, despite the large proportion whose cause of death was directly attributable to substance abuse.

References

1. P. W. Haberman and M. M. Baden, "Drinking, Drugs and Death," *International Journal of the Addictions 9:* 1974, pp. 761–73.
2. E. M. Brecher and eds., "The 'Heroin Overdose' Mystery and Other Occupational Hazards of Addiction," in: *The Consumer's Union Report: Licit and Illicit Drugs*, Boston: Little, Brown, 1972, pp. 101–14.
3. *McKinney's Consolidated Laws of New York*, Vehicle and Traffic Law, 62A; Section 1192, as amended in 1972, St. Paul, Minn.: West Publishing, Suppl. 1972–1973.
4. P. W. Haberman, "Differences Between Families Admitting and Denying an Existing Drinking Problem," *Journal of Health and Human Behavior 4:* 1963, pp. 141–45.
5. See for example D. Cahalan, *Problem Drinkers*, San Francisco: Jossey-Bass, 1970; H. A. Mulford, "Drinking and Deviant Drinking, U.S.A., 1963," *Quarterly Journal of Studies on Alcohol 25:* 1964, pp. 634–50, M. B. Bailey, P. W. Haberman, and H. Alksne, "The Epidemiology of Alcoholism in an Urban Residential Area," *Quarterly Journal of Studies on Alcohol 26:* 1965, pp. 19–40; P. W. Haberman and J. Sheinberg, "Implicative Drinking Reported in a Household Survey," *Quarterly Journal of Studies on Alcohol 28:* 1967, pp. 538–43.
6. C. P. Larson, "Alcohol: Fact and Fallacy," in: *Legal Medicine Annual, 1969,* C. H. Wecht, ed., New York: Appleton-Century-Crofts, 1969, pp. 239–68.
7. Adapted from Table 5 in J. N. Cross, *Guide to the Community Control of Alcoholism*, New York: American Public Health Association, 1968, p. 22.
8. M. M. Baden and D. J. Ottenberg, "Alcohol—The All-American Drug of Choice," L. London, mod., *Contemporary Drug Problems, A Law Quarterly 6:* 1974, pp. 101–25.
9. C. Cherubin et al., "The Epidemiology of Death in Narcotic Addicts," *American Journal of Epidemiology 96:* 1972, pp. 11–22.
10. P. W. Haberman, "The Reliability and Validity of the Data," in *Poverty*

and Health: A Sociological Analysis, J. Kosa, A. Antonovsky, and I. K. Zola, eds., Cambridge, Mass.: Harvard University Press, 1969, pp. 343–83.

11. G. Beall and S. Cobb, "The Frequency Distribution of Episodes of Rheumatoid Arthritis as Shown by Periodic Examination," *Journal of Chronic Diseases 14:* 1961, pp. 291–310.

12. L. Breslow, editorial in *Journal of Chronic Diseases 14:* 1961, pp. 289–90.

4

Multiple Drug Use

A recent National Institute on Drug Abuse (NIDA) publication states that "a majority of drug users, from the junior high school experimenter to the hard-core narcotic addict, employ more than one legal or illegal substance to alter their subjective states (1)." Three major categories of patterns of multiple drug use are described: (a) combinations of either ethical fixed-drug preparations or illicit mixtures; (b) separate drugs taken concomitantly; and (c) two or more substances taken sequentially or consecutively.

Amphetamine-barbiturate mixtures such as Dexamyl and heroin combined with cocaine ("speedballs") are examples of the combination-type of multiple drug use (1). In addition, many street drugs contain unknown additives and impurities which have no psychopharmacological (mood-altering) effects but do contribute to medical complications. Two common examples of concomitant multiple drug use are Quaaludes (methaqualone) taken together with alcohol to enhance the depressant action of each compound, and amphetamines with barbiturates to counter the restlessness, insomnia, and excitation produced by the amphetamines.

Different substances may be used sequentially, both medically and nonmedically, to control the time span of a drug-induced state. Perhaps the most familiar example of this pattern is the alternate use of medically prescribed barbiturates in the evening for sleep and amphetamines, often prescribed for weight loss, in the morning for alertness and energy. This pattern involves the improper use of prescribed drugs by adults as a coping mechanism and should be distinguished from the illegal use of such drugs, especially by adolescents, for their euphoric effects. It is the latter type of abuse that is associated with unnatural death.

Newspapers and other media, it should be noted, have tended to overstate the fatal consequences of multiple drug use. Such reactions are very unlikely to occur as a result of casual or inadvertent ingestion of one or two extra pills and/or drinks containing alcohol. The multiple drug users seen at the Medical Examiner's Office are primarily chronic abusers who took much more than a medically indicated quantity of pills.

If the user's drug of choice is unobtainable, other drugs may be substituted for it. Thus narcotics addicts are likely to become heavy users of barbiturates and/or alcohol temporarily, in an attempt to alleviate withdrawal symptoms when heroin is not available. Likewise, when there is a scarcity of the illicit drug of choice, the addict may use it sequentially or concomitantly with other drugs, to reduce or ration his use of the scarce drug.

Multiple drug use can also be categorized according to pharmacological classes of the substances. The drug abuser often restricts himself to a single category of substances, namely the depressants (alcohol, narcotics, sedatives, and tranquilizers), the stimulants (amphetamines and cocaine), or the hallucinogens (marijuana, LSD, and related substances).

Depressants, more than other groups of mood-altering substances such as stimulants and hallucinogens are potentially life threatening. Thus, multiple drug use among our Medical Examiner population consisted primarily of concomitant, and possible sequential, use of depressants. Positive findings of combination and concomitant use can be obtained by means of toxicologic tests, but sequential use is not likely to be revealed by postmortem medical procedures due to the time span between the use of different substances.

In order to obtain the data required for analyzing multiple use of mood-altering drugs among decedents, we coded drugs (including alcohol) according to their pharmacological class. This procedure is similar to the methods Lerner and Nurco used in their study of drug abuse deaths in Baltimore (2).

The code categories for mood-altering drugs developed for our study are based on postmortem findings and the method of recording such findings. Our code categories are: heroin, morphine, or other opiates; methadone; hypnotics and sedatives (mainly barbiturates); tranquilizers (both minor and major ones); Darvon (propoxyphene); cocaine; and alcohol.

Therefore, our sample in this chapter is limited, for the most part, to those decedents on whom a blood or brain alcohol concentration (BAC) and toxicologic tests for recent use of other drugs were performed. Toxicologic findings were obtained for 1429 persons, 73 percent of the total sample, including 10 (0.5%) for whom no BAC was obtained, so that those 518 cases that were missing both postmortem medical procedures are excluded from much of this analysis. In seven additional cases (0.4%), a BAC was performed, but no postmortem tests for other drugs were performed. Since the presence or absence of only one drug, alcohol, was tested, these seven cases also are only partially analyzed. For purposes of our study, alcohol toxicology is referred to as BAC and is distinguished from toxicologic analyses for all other mood-altering drugs. The term "toxicology" is used to refer to drugs other than alcohol.

Among the drugs of abuse, alcohol is most easily detected and quantitated in postmortem tests, and is metabolized similarly in all people at a relatively constant rate (3). The brain alcohol level is virtually the same as the blood alcohol level. Because of technical problems in obtaining accurate postmortem blood samples, brain analysis may be preferable for medicolegal purposes. Blood and brain alcohol concentrations are used interchangeably in our study.

As mentioned in Chapter 2, heroin is rapidly metabolized to morphine, which is the drug usually detected in heroin addicts. There is considerable individual variability in the metabolism of other drugs, except for barbiturates, so that quantitation is not as meaningful. Therefore, we recorded only the presence or absence, not the quantity, of drugs other than alcohol found in postmortem tests. For alcohol, as previously indicated, the specific concentration was obtained. There are at present no routine toxicologic tests for some other drugs such as marijuana, LSD, and other hallucinogens (4,5). Low levels of amphetamines are also difficult to detect toxicologically, and amphetamine overdose has very rarely been recorded as a cause of death (6).

Use and Abuse of Specific Drugs

The data on the use of specific mood-altering drugs in our sample come from two different sources and reflect different aspects of drug use. Informants were likely to report the decedents' drug of choice as the cause of related problems, suggesting chronic substance abuse. Positive toxicologic findings in our sample generally indicated recent use before death by chronic abusers of their drug of choice and/or substitutes. However, a few of these decedents with positive toxicologic findings were only occasional users or experimenters, and others had used pills to commit suicide.

Overall, 28 percent of the decedents were reported by informants to have had some problem because of drug use and multiple drug use was indicated by 8 percent of the informants. Heroin (20.2%) was mentioned by informants much more often than any other drug; barbiturates (5.8%) and illicitly used methadone (2.2%) were the only others reported by more than one percent. Heroin caused drug-related problems that were perceived by informants in a slightly larger proportion than the 20.2 percent reported since 1.8 percent of those with problems due to unknown drugs (3.2%) had toxicologic findings of narcotics use. In addition, a greater proportion of decedents than was indicated by informants probably had drug problems due to illicit methadone use since the small percentage (2.2%) does not include any use by decedents who were reported to be in methadone maintenance treatment programs (MMTP). It could not be determined whether methadone use reported for patients in treatment programs included illicit as well as maintenance doses. Very few decedents were reported to have had problems because of cocaine, LSD, amphetamine, tranquilizer, or marijuana use. The use of marijuana in particular may very well have been widespread in this sample, but related problems were likely to be trivial in comparison to those caused by heroin addiction.

Table 4–1. Decedents' Use of Mood-Altering Drugs Revealed in Toxicologic Findings

MOOD-ALTERING DRUGS	TOXICOLOGIC FINDINGS N = 1429[a]	
	Alone or Combination (Percent Using Drugs)	*Sum for Each Drug (Percent Using Drug)*
Morphine (heroin metabolite) and methadone	3.7%	—
Morphine and other drug(s)[b]	2.0	—
Methadone and other drug(s)	6.6	—
Hypnotics (mostly barbiturates; including sedatives) and other drugs[c]	3.6	—
Morphine alone	7.0[d]	(12.7%)
Methadone alone	6.5	(16.8)
Hypnotics alone	4.8	(11.5)
Tranquilizers alone	5.3	(12.3)
Darvon (propoxyphene)[e] alone	1.5	(4.0)
Cocaine alone	0.5	(1.0)
Other	0.8[f]	(0.8)
Total	42.3%	(59.1%)

a. Proportion with toxicology obtained is 73.1% of total N of 1954.

b. With or without other listed mood-altering drugs.

c. With subsequent listed mood-altering drug(s).

d. Includes 16 (1.1%) with toxicologic findings of quinine or lidocaine, and narcotics use implicated elsewhere.

e. Darvon is similar to narcotics, but does not have their analgesic potency and is considered herein as a non-narcotic, mood-altering drug.

f. Includes 8 (0.6%) that were classified as narcotics abusers and had narcotism certified as cause of death.

Toxicologic findings of mood-altering drugs are presented in Table 4.1. In total, 42 percent of the decedents who had toxicologic tests had used some mood-altering substance shortly before death and 17 percent of them had evidence of multiple drug use. Methadone was found in 17 percent of the toxicologic tests. Three other depressants—morphine (the heroin metabolite) (12.7%), tranquilizers (12.3%), and barbiturates (11.5%)—were also found in more than 10 percent of the toxicologies. While morphine was the drug most frequently found alone in the postmortem testing (7.0%), methadone was the one most often used concomitantly with non-narcotic drugs (10.3%). Concomitant use of the two narcotics, heroin and methadone, shortly before death represented a substantial portion (3.7%) of the multiple drug use. Darvon (4.0%) and cocaine (1.0%) were the only other mood-altering substances present in any appreciable number of cases.

There was a strong positive relationship between the specific types of drugs reported by informants and those found in toxicologic tests (see Table 4.2). Seventy-one percent of the decedents classified by informants as narcotics abusers showed toxicologic evidence of recent narcotics use. As previously mentioned, decedents reported to have had problems with unspecified drugs more often than not were probably narcotics abusers since more than half (52.0%) had narcotics in their system at the time of death. For 42 percent of those reported to have had problems with non-narcotic drugs, primarily barbiturates, there were toxicologic findings of such drugs, and 8 percent of them had used narcotics just before death. On the other hand, 73 percent of those reported to have had no drug problems also showed no postmortem evidence of drug use.

The BAC and other toxicologic findings for all decedents according to their classification as alcoholics, narcotics abusers, those with both conditions, and nonabusers are presented in Table 4.3. Positive

Table 4–2. Toxicologic Findings According to Drug Problems as Reported by Informants

USE ACCORDING TO TOXICOLOGIC FINDINGS		DRUGS REPORTED BY INFORMANTS TO CAUSE PROBLEMS		
	N:	Narcotics (331)[b]	Unspecified Drug(s) (50)[b]	Other Mood-altering Drug(s)[a] (36)[b]	None (1011)[b]
Narcotics		71.0%	52.0%	8.3%	10.3%
Other mood-altering drug(s) only[c]		10.0	22.0	41.7	16.4
Negative		19.0	26.0	50.0	73.3
Total		100%	100%	100%	100%

a. Primarily (59.1%) barburates.

b. Total N and proportions with toxicology obtained are: narcotics 398 and 83.2%; unspecified drugs 63 and 79.4%; other mood-altering drugs 44 and 81.8%; none 1449 and 69.8%.

c. Primarily hypnotics (mostly barbiturates) and/or tranquilizers.

Table 4–3. BAC and Other Toxicology for Decedents According to Classification as Alcoholics and/or Narcotics Abusers

BAC AND OTHER TOXICOLOGY[a]	ALL DECEDENTS	ALCOHOLICS	NARCOTICS ABUSERS	BOTH CONDITIONS	NON-ABUSERS
N:	(1429)[b]	(316)[b]	(305)[b]	(181)[b]	(627)[b]
Other toxicology negative					
BAC negative[c]	32.3%	29.4%	7.2%	6.6%	53.4%
BAC .01 – .09%	8.8	13.6	3.3	4.4	10.4
BAC .10% or above	17.4	36.4	4.3	8.3	16.7
BAC negative[d]					
Morphine (heroin metabolite) and methadone	2.4	n.a.*	8.5	4.4	n.a.
Morphine	6.1	n.a.	22.3	10.5	n.a.
Methadone	9.5	n.a.	32.5	20.4	n.a.
Other mood-altering drugs only	9.4	7.6	4.3	6.6	13.7
BAC positive					
Morphine and methadone	1.3	n.a.	3.0	5.5	n.a.
Morphine	2.9	n.a.	6.2	12.2	n.a.
Methadone	3.6	n.a.	7.5	15.5	n.a.
Other mood-altering drugs only	6.3	13.0	1.0	5.5	5.7
Total	100%	100%	100%	100%	100%

a. Toxicology categories for drugs other than alcohol:
Negative – no mood-altering drugs present.
Morphine (heroin metabolite) and methadone – with or without other mood-altering drug(s).
Morphine – no methadone, but with or without other mood-altering drug(s).
Methadone – no morphine, but with or without other mood-altering drug(s).
Other mood-altering drugs only – primarily (87.6%) hypnotics (mostly barbiturates) and/or tranquilizers.

b. Total N and proportions with toxicologies obtained are: all decedents 1954 and 73.1%; alcoholics 581 and 54.4%; narcotics abusers 339 and 90.0%; both conditions 222 and 81.5%; nonabusers 812 and 77.2%.

c. Includes 6 (0.3%) with BAC not obtained.

d. Includes 4 (0.2%) with BAC not obtained.

* n.a. – not applicable.

BACs were naturally most common among alcoholics – followed in order by those with both conditions, nonabusers, and narcotics abusers. Sixty-three percent of the alcoholics, 51 percent of those with both conditions, 33 percent of the nonabusers, and 25 percent of the narcotics abusers had alcohol in their system at the time of death. The proportions for these substance abuse groups with alcohol concentrations of 0.10 percent or above, indicating impairment or intoxication, were in the same order: alcoholics (44.6%), those with both conditions (30.9%), nonabusers (19.3%), and narcotics abusers (11.1%). Thus, a majority of decedents with positive BACs in all groups, except for those classified as narcotics abusers, had sufficiently elevated alcohol levels to have had impaired judgement and coordination. The alcoholics were also those most likely to have used alcohol and other non-narcotic drugs concomitantly (13.0%).

A substantial proportion of the nonabusers who took other mood-altering drugs before death were suicide victims, primarily by an overdose of pills. Suicide by taking pills, usually barbiturates or other hypnotics, does not have the long-term implications of chronic abuse for purposes of euphoria as present in narcotics addicts.

Among narcotics abusers who were also classified as alcoholics, 35 percent had used only narcotics just before death; 33 percent had used narcotics in combination with alcohol; and 19 percent had used only alcohol. Sixty-three percent of the narcotics abusers not classified as alcoholics showed toxicologic evidence of narcotics alone, so that multiple drug use including alcohol was much less likely to be related to their deaths. Among all narcotics abusers, methadone (49.3%) was found in toxicologic tests more often than morphine (37.2%). Comparable proportions had postmortem evidence of alcohol use in combination with methadone (14.4%) or morphine (12.4%). For 11 percent of all narcotics abusers, there were toxicologic findings of concomitant heroin and methadone use.

Heroin and Methadone "Overdose" Deaths

There has been much recent publicity about the true nature of heroin deaths, often mislabeled as being due to "overdose" (7). Earlier data from the New York City Chief Medical Examiner's Office gave several indications that many of these narcotics deaths were not caused by pharmacological overdose (8,9). Toxicologic tests on dead addicts, and on drugs found at the scene of death, rarely reveal evidence of more than usual concentrations of heroin, roughly 5 mg in a packet.

Second, almost all of those who died of alleged overdoses were chronic, long-term addicts who had developed a tolerance for large amounts of heroin rather than recent unaddicted experimenters. Finally, more than one death among addicts using the same heroin supply was rare.

Alternate explanations of these deaths are multiple drug use including alcohol, acute reaction to an adulterant or diluent of heroin, and the unsterile manner in which drugs are taken. It is often overlooked that about 95 percent of the ingredients in a packet of "street" heroin are unsterile, frequently unknown adulterants, in unknown quantities. Quinine, the most common adulterant of heroin in New York City, has been noted to cause rapid death with pulmonary edema, similar to heroin (7). The concomitant use of heroin with alcohol and/or other depressants, such as barbiturates, has a synergistic or additive effect that may also be fatal. Deaths related to methadone use are usually due to true pharmacological overdoses taken by persons who obtain illicit methadone and have not gradually been made tolerant to maintenance doses; such doses may contain 20 times more narcotics predissolved in juice (100 mg in high-maintenance daily doses) as in a packet of "street" heroin (10). Deaths may also be due to taking methadone concomitantly with other drugs of abuse. Persons have died while in official custody during withdrawal from methadone, as well as from alcohol (delirium tremens) and barbiturates, but not from heroin withdrawal.

Since heroin is metabolized rapidly to morphine in the body, toxicologic findings of quinine or lidocaine—the only other common adulterant for heroin which can be routinely identified toxicologically—suggest that heroin was used (10). When toxicologic evidence of morphine was found in our study, the narcotic used was almost always heroin and the presence of adulterants was not recorded. The toxicologic findings in Table 4.4 do implicate the concomitant use of alcohol and/or other mood-altering drugs by many of the persons whose deaths were attributed to narcotism. One-half (49.5%) of them showed toxicologic evidence of both narcotics and other mood-altering substances. Methadone was present in a considerably larger proportion of deaths (66.8%) than morphine (39.4%), particularly in combination with alcohol and/or other drugs. Methadone was found with other mood-altering substances in more than twice as many

Table 4–4. Toxicology when Cause of Death Was Certified as Narcotism[a]

TOXICOLOGY	NARCOTISM DEATHS $(N = 226)$[b]
Morphine (heroin metabolite) and methadone	11.1%
Morphine and methadone with alcohol and/or other (mood-altering) drugs	4.9
Morphine with alcohol and/or other drugs	11.9
Morphine only	11.5
Methadone with alcohol and/or other drugs	32.7
Methadone only	18.1
Other[c]	9.7
Total	100%

a. Without alcoholism.
b. Total N and proportion with toxicology obtained are 247 and 91.5%.
c. Toxicology negative for morphine (heroin metabolite) or methadone.

cases (37.6%) as was heroin (16.8%). Finally, it should be pointed out that 16 percent had evidence of both heroin and methadone use just before death.

In our sample, 151 persons 18 years of age or older whose cause of death was certified as narcotism had toxicologic evidence of methadone. Since about one-half of the drug deaths investigated by the Medical Examiner's Office from August 20, 1974 to August 19, 1975 were in our sample, approximately 300 narcotism deaths involving methadone occurred during that twelve-month period. Methadone was precent in about two-thirds of adults whose deaths were directly due to taking narcotics.

Postmortem Toxicologic Findings in Methadone Treatment Evaluation

Methadone maintenance has expanded greatly from the first experiment by Dole and Nyswander in 1965 (11), and has now become the major treatment for heroin addiction. Theoretically it acts by blocking the pleasurable effects of heroin. Advantages of methadone over heroin maintenance are that it can be taken effectively by mouth and is long-lasting, requiring only one dose a day. Methadone is a synthetic narcotic and thus produces cross-tolerance to heroin, differing from narcotics antagonists such as cyclazocine and naloxene in two major respects. Although these antagonists also block the pleasurable effects of heroin, unlike methadone, they are not addicting and patients can and do stop taking them at will and become readdicted to heroin. Furthermore antagonists do not alleviate postaddiction anxiety, depression, and craving as methadone does (12).

The original results of methadone treatment, evaluated by Gearing (13), showed that most patients remained in treatment and that their illicit drug use and arrest rates declined. They also became much more socially responsible and economically productive. In recent years, however, many programs have failed to reproduce these early favorable results with resultant criticism of methadone treatment programs lately. Although the method of administering methadone has not changed significantly, many other aspects of the programs are now different. The recent mixed results have been attributed variously to changes in the treatment clinic staffs, treatment procedures or styles, admisisions criteria, and in the addict population. The first patients were older than more recent ones, and had no history of alcoholism, multiple drug use, or mental disorder. Addicts are now younger, more likely to be abusers of alcohol or other drugs, and thus may be more difficult to treat successfully by any method. Furthermore, as methadone treatment has expanded, intensive psychological and social services have been curtailed, and the patient load for maintenance clinic staff has increased greatly.

It has been shown that multiple drug use is a fairly common occurrence among heroin addicts enrolled in methadone maintenance (or narcotics antagonist) programs (1,14). After addicts have been stabilized on methadone so that the pleasurable effects of heroin may no longer be attained, they frequently abuse alcohol and barbiturates. Multidrug abuse involving mainly alcohol and barbiturates has been viewed as the most prevalent and serious complication of methadone maintenance treatment for a number of reasons (1,15–17). Multiple-drug users tend to be more resistant to treatment and to have more complications and poorer prognoses than single-drug users. Of particular relevance to our cases, withdrawal from barbiturates or alcohol is much more life-threatening than heroin withdrawal. In addition, because of the synergistic effect of different types of depressants, the use of barbiturates, tranquilizers, and/or alcohol concomitantly with methadone or heroin increases the risk of death as compared to the use of narcotics alone.

Because of the growing controversy over methadone maintenance of heroin addicts, we have examined the multiple use of narcotics, alcohol, and other mood-altering drugs just before death, according to whether or not the narcotics abusers were reported to have been in a methadone maintenance program. Informants who reported that persons in our sample had a problem because of narcotics use were also asked if the decedent was in a methadone program. The patient status of questionable cases was verified by the Methadone Maintenance Evaluation Unit of the Columbia University School of Public Health (18), utilizing data from Rockefeller University. Unfortunately, we do not have any information on the methadone treatment status of these patients at the time of death—and some may have dropped out of the program. Also, no questions were asked about any other treatment such as residence in drug-free therapeutic communities. With these limitations, the data recorded in Table 4.5 describe the multiple drug-use patterns just before death of heroin addicts according to their status in methadone maintenance treatment programs.

Multiple use of alcohol (19,20) and/or other drugs (1,21,22) by heroin addicts before methadone or other treatment has also been well documented. Among the narcotics abusers in our sample whose MMTP status was reported by informants, similar proportions of patients and nonpatients had postmortem evidence of concomitant alcohol and/or other drug use. In fact, Table 4.5 shows that those narcotics abusers who had not been patients were somewhat more likely to have had positive BACs than were those in MMTP. Forty-five percent of the nonpatients and 34 percent of the patients had postmortem evidence of alcohol use. The proportions that had used only non-narcotic mood-altering drugs just before death were 9.8 percent for nonpatients and 10.1 percent for patients.

Several other postmortem findings for these MMTP patients and nonpatients are also noteworthy. Twice as many untreated narcotics abusers (18.8%) as patients (9.5%) had only alcohol in their system at the time of death. Although the same proportion of both groups had toxicologic evidence of morphine (patients 31.0%; nonpatients

Table 4-5. BAC and Other Toxicology for Informant-Classified Narcotics Abusers According to Reported Methadone Maintenance Treatment Program (MMTP) Status

BAC AND OTHER TOXICOLOGY[a]	N:	MMTP STATUS	
		Patients (219)[b]	*Nonpatients* (112)[b]
Other toxicology negative			
BAC negative		5.5%[c]	8.9%
BAC .01–.09%		3.6	7.1
BAC .10% or above		5.9	10.7
BAC negative			
Morphine (heroin metabolite) and methadone		7.8	7.1
Morphine		14.1	13.4
Methadone		32.9[c]	17.0
Other mood-altering drugs only		5.5	8.9[d]
BAC positive			
Morphine and methadone		2.7	5.4
Morphine		6.4	7.1
Methadone		11.0	13.4
Other mood-altering drugs only		4.6	0.9
Total		100%	100%

a. Toxicology categories for drugs other than alcohol:
Negative — no mood-altering drugs present.
Morphine (heroin metabolite) and methadone — with or without other mood-altering drug(s).
Morphine — no methadone, but with or without other mood-altering drug(s).
Methadone — no morphine, but with or without other mood-altering drug(s).
Other mood-altering drugs only — primarily barbiturates and/or tranquilizers.
b. Total N and proportions with toxicologies obtained are: patients 269 and 81.4%; nonpatients 129 and 86.8%.
c. Includes 1 (0.5%) with BAC not obtained.
d. Includes 1 (0.9%) with BAC not obtained.

33.0%), methadone was found, as anticipated, in a larger proportion of patients (54.4%) than nonpatients (42.9%). Thus more than one-half of the patients had methadone in their system at the time of death, including 13 percent without postmortem evidence of alcohol or other drugs, but we do not know the extent to which these postmortem findings of methadone exceeded the maintenance treatment doses. In addition, comparable proportions of these patients and nonpatients (50.2% and 45.8%, respectively) died directly of narcotism.

A study of methadone related deaths which was conducted at the Medical Examiner's Office during the same time period as our study provides some additional data on methadone use by our sample (23). In the study, persons with toxicologic findings of methadone, including those who died as a result of trauma and of drug-taking directly, were divided into three groups—nonpatients, previous patients, or current patients—according to their MMTP status at the time of death. Previous patients were those whose patient status had been terminated, voluntarily or involuntarily, because of about two weeks' absence or more without advance authorization, or those who had been expelled as required by the Food and Drug Administration's regulations (24). Of the 217 cases in both studies, all of whom had methadone present at death, 46 percent were nonpatients, 23 percent were previous patients, and 31 percent were current patients. The nonpatients and previous patients were using methadone illicitly, and some current patients presumably had taken more than their daily maintenance doses. Informants were much more likely to admit that former or current MMTP patients, rather than nonpatients, had problems because of narcotics use. Ninety-three percent of the 118 patients, but only 44 percent of the 99 nonpatients, were reported to have had problems due to narcotics.

A substantial minority of MMTP patients did not have evidence of recently prescribed methadone use prior to death. This may account for some deaths of MMTP patients who lose tolerance, perhaps because they sell or give away their take-home supply and then die after taking a dose to which they had been previously tolerant. Methadone is detectable in body tissues and fluids for many days after last usage (23). But, toxicologic tests can only reveal the presence of methadone, not the degree of tolerance or illicit increments taken.

This evidence of widespread use of illicit methadone by nonpatients and of heroin by MMTP patients in our Medical Examiner population is striking. Since methadone is to be taken daily, patients who cannot come to a clinic every day must be trusted with "take-home" doses, some of which are used illicitly by nonpatients. Patients, presumably stabilized on methadone, may take heroin sporadically to test the blocking action of methadone, or heroin may be

used for euphoria when their methadone dose is losing its effectiveness. The blocking effect of methadone varies directly with the
dosage, so that a larger dose of methadone will block a larger quantity
of heroin (12). In any interpretation of our results, for the purpose of
MMTP evaluation it must be emphasized that cases such as ours are
one type of program failure, not all of which had been previously
recognized as failures. Furthermore, 82 percent of those reported to
have had problems due to drug use had their most recent trouble
within the year before they died, suggesting that many were not enrolled in MMTP at the time of death.

During the twelve-month period beginning August 20, 1974 when
our sample was obtained, there was a daily average of approximately
28,000 active MMTP patients enrolled in 119 clinics (240 patients per
clinic) located in the Bronx, Manhattan, Queens, or Staten Island. The
Office of Chief Medical Examiner investigated 600 or so deaths of
MMTP patients during that twelve-month period (including the 269
in our sample reported to have been in MMTP) which was equal to
about 2 percent of the patient population in these four boroughs.
However, the death rate for all adults in the same age group as most
MMTP patients (18 to 39 years) is roughly 0.2 percent or one-tenth
the rate for patients.

Characteristics of Different Substance Abusers

Selected demographic and health characteristics of decedents classified as alcoholics, narcotics abusers, and those with both conditions
are shown in Table 4.6. The characteristics were chosen and grouped
so as to best describe the differences and similarities among these
subgroups. In demographic terms, the alcoholics differed markedly
from the narcotics abusers and those with both conditions. The proportion of whites was highest among the alcoholics. Alcoholics were
much older than decedents in the other subgroups, most often had
only a grade school education, and had been currently or previously
married.

Hispanic and black substance abusers in our sample were grouped
according to their place of birth — Puerto Rico or elsewhere for the
Hispanics, southern states and New York City or elsewhere for the

blacks. White substance abusers were grouped according to their religion at the time of death as Catholics, Protestants, and Jews. We
had a sufficiently large number of Catholics to categorize them as
native-born and foreign-born. Blacks who were alcoholics were most
often from the South, while blacks who were narcotics abusers or had
both conditions were mainly born in New York City. Among the
whites, Protestants and foreign-born Catholics were much more frequently alcoholics than narcotics abusers, whereas slightly larger
proportions of narcotics abusers were native-born Catholics and
Jews. The alcoholics were on average twenty years older than the
narcotics abusers and fourteen years older than those with both conditions. The generation gap between the alcoholics and others ac-
counts for the difference in their final marital status and perhaps in
their educational attainment.

The principal activity of these decedents during their last year of
life clearly demonstrates the social problems associated with substance abuse. Less than two-fifths in each subgroup had been working for most of the year preceding their death, even though four-
fifths were men. Only among the alcoholics was there more than one
person who had reached retirement age. Twenty-six percent of those
with both conditions and 22 percent of the alcoholics had been sick
most of the past year. Indeed, 92 percent of the 446 alcoholics classified as such by informants had a problem—most often with their
health—due to drinking within a year of death. Furthermore, 80
percent of the 175 who received help did so within their last year of
life, and 51 percent did so at a hospital. Twenty-seven percent of
those with both conditions, 25 percent of the narcotics abusers, and
14 percent of the alcoholics had been doing nothing during most of
the last year except drinking, taking drugs, or spending time in jail.

There has been considerable speculation about a possible increase
in narcotics use because of what has been described as "the heroin
addiction epidemic among American soldiers in Vietnam in 1970 and
1971 (25)." Fifty-four percent of 82 men in our sample who served
during the Vietnam War were classified as narcotics abusers. They
comprise 15.1 percent of all the male narcotics abusers and 10.5 percent of those with both conditions who were eligible for service during the Vietnam War. A larger proportion, (about 22 percent) of all
eligible men living in New York City were veterans of the Vietnam

Table 4–6. Characteristics of Decedents According to Classification as Alcoholics and/or Narcotics Abusers

CHARACTERISTICS	ALCOHOLICS	NARCOTICS ABUSERS	BOTH CONDITIONS
N:	(581)	(339)	(222)
Sex			
Male	78.0%	83.5%	80.6%
Ethnicity[a]			
Hispanic[b]			
Birthplace Puerto Rico	13.6%	15.0%	18.9%
Birthplace New York City	4.8	6.8	9.0
or elsewhere[c]	(18.4)	(21.8)	(27.9)
Black			
Birthplace southern states[d]	26.9	10.6	15.8
Birthplace New York City	12.1	34.8	35.1
or elsewhere[e]	(39.0)	(45.4)	(50.9)
White			
Catholic, native-born	19.5	21.3	14.0
Catholic, foreign-born	6.2	1.8	0.4
Jewish	2.1	4.4	1.8
Protestant[f]	14.8	5.3	5.0
	(42.6)	(32.8)	(21.2)
Total	100%	100%	100%
Age at last birthday			
18–29	9.5%	72.0%	42.3%
30–49	50.4	26.2	51.4
50 or older	40.1	1.8	6.3
Total	100%	100%	100%
Median age	46 yrs.	26 yrs.	32 yrs.
Education			
Grade school or none	23.6%	11.2%	15.4%
Some high school	22.4	44.5	44.1
High school graduate	25.3	28.9	24.8
Some college, or more	13.9	13.6	8.1
Unknown	14.8	1.8	7.7
Total	100%	100%	100%
Marital status			
Never married	28.9%	63.4%	57.7%
Married[g]	30.5	20.1	19.8
Previously married	40.0	16.5	21.3
Unknown	0.7	—	1.4
Total	100%	100%	100%
Principal activity in past year			
Working	36.7%	37.5%	24.3%
Sick	21.7	8.3	26.1

Table 4-6. Continued

CHARACTERISTICS	ALCOHOLICS	NARCOTICS ABUSERS	BOTH CONDITIONS
N:	(581)	(339)	(222)
Drinking, taking drugs, nothing, jail	14.4	25.4	27.1
Retired	9.8	0.3	0.5
Other, unknown	17.3	28.6	22.1
Total	100%	100%	100%
Armed Forces Services (men, age 20-36)[h]	(115)	(218)	(105)
Vietnam War	10.4%	15.1%	10.5%
MMTP patients	n.a.*	41.9%	57.2%
Hospitalization for liver trouble			
Probably due to alcohol	13.6%	0.6%	16.2%
Hepatitis, probably related to heroin use	0.9%	13.9%	7.7%
Cause-of-death certification			
Natural	7.2%	1.8%	0.5%
Accident[i]	17.0	5.0	5.9
Suicide	10.5	7.1	4.5
Homicide	18.2	31.6	17.6
Substance abuse[j]	47.0	54.6	71.6
Total	100%	100%	100%

a. Excludes one Oriental alcoholic.

b. Decedent or at least one parent born in Puerto Rico or Spanish-speaking country in Western Hemisphere, irrespective of color.

c. 56.3% born in New York City, remainder born outside United States in Western Hemisphere.

d. Southern States are Alabama, Arkansas, Delaware, District of Columbia, Florida, Georgia, Kentucky, Louisiana, Maryland, Mississippi, Oklahoma, North Carolina, South Carolina, Tennessee, Texas, Virginia, and West Virginia.

e. 80.8% born in New York City, 94.7% in United States.

f. Includes other, none, or unknown religion.

g. Includes 18.0% in common-law marriages.

h. Question added to interview 9/5/74 after 94 (4.8%) cases done. Men age 20 to 36 in 1975 were age-eligible for draft during Vietnam War (age 18 to 26 in period 1964 to 1973).

i. Includes less than 1% in each subgroup who died of accidental poisoning from drugs other than alcohol or narcotics.

j. Alcoholism and/or narcotism alone or with other cause of death.

* n.a. = not applicable.

War (26). Furthermore, almost as large a proportion of eligible men in our sample who were alcoholics (10.4%) and nonabusers (10.1%) were also Vietnam War veterans. It should also be noted that these men in our sample were in the age, ethnic, and socioeconomic groups most vulnerable to heroin addiction, and they lived in an area where illicit drugs were relatively easy to obtain.

With regard to the health characteristics in Table 4.6, decedents who were classified as both narcotics abusers and alcoholics had more often been MMTP patients than those classified only as narcotics abusers. Forty-eight percent of all the narcotics abusers — including 57 percent of those with both conditions and 42 percent of those classified as narcotics abusers only — were reported to have received methadone maintenance treatment. Those decedents with both conditions had been hospitalized for liver trouble (probably due to alcohol) somewhat more often than the pure alcoholics, and were much closer statistically to the narcotics abusers in the proportion hospitalized for hepatitis (probably due to heroin use). As mentioned in Chapter 3, substance abuse itself was the major cause of death in all three subgroups and was especially predominant among those with both conditions. The proportion that died as a result of accidents, suicide, and natural causes was highest among the alcoholics. Homicide was a much more frequent cause of death among narcotics abusers, although large proportions in the other two subgroups were also homicide victims.

The characteristics of decedents classified as alcoholics, narcotics abusers, and those with both conditions are remarkably similar to those in our 1972 pilot study (27). Our conclusions from these pilot study data that decedents with both conditions were almost always primarily narcotics abusers who also abused alcohol (rather than alcoholics who had become narcotics addicts), have been confirmed by the findings in our main study. In the two studies, those with both conditions resembled the narcotics abusers much more than the alcoholics demographically; they differed from the narcotics abusers mainly in that they were older. In the main study, those with both conditions, showed evidence of physical damage due to alcohol abuse almost as often as did the alcoholics. There was physical evidence of alcoholism in 86 percent of 506 alcoholics and in 76 percent of 207 persons with both conditions upon whom autopsies were performed.

Summary

With regard to the use and abuse of specific drugs by our sample, methadone, morphine (the heroin metabolite), tranquilizers, and barbiturates (in that order) were each found in at least 10 percent of the toxicologic tests, whereas only heroin was mentioned by more than 5 percent of the informants. The concomitant use of alcohol and/or other mood-altering drugs was implicated, not only in deaths attributed to narcotism, but in other unnatural and violent deaths as well. Methadone, was found more often than morphine in toxicologic tests on persons who died of narcotism. There was toxicologic evidence of widespread heroin use by MMTP patients and illicit methadone use by nonpatients in our sample. Narcotics abusers who were also classified as alcoholics were older than (but otherwise similar to) other narcotics abusers, and had physical evidence of chronic alcohol abuse.

References

1. National Clearinghouse for Drug Abuse Information, NIDA, *Polydrug Use: An Annotated Bibliography*, Washington, D.C.: DHEW Publication No. (ADM) 1975, pp. 75–225.
2. M. Lerner and D. N. Nurco, "Drug Abuse Deaths in Baltimore, 1951–1966," *International Journal of the Addictions 5:* 1970, pp. 693–715.
3. C. P. Larson, "Alcohol: Fact and Fallacy," in: *Legal Medicine Annual, 1969*, C. H. Wecht, ed., New York: Appleton-Century-Crofts, 1969, pp. 239–68.
4. M. M. Baden, "Narcotic Abuse: A Medical Examiner's View," *New York State Journal of Medicine 72:* 1972, pp. 834–40.
5. M. M. Baden et al., "Detection of Drugs of Abuse in Urine," in *Medical Aspects of Drug Abuse*, R. W. Richter, ed., Hagerstown, Md.: Harper & Row, 1975, pp. 72–78.
6. J. C. Kramer, "Introduction to Amphetamine Use," in: *Current Concepts on Amphetamine Abuse*, E. H. Ellinwood and S. Cohen, eds., Washington, D. C.: U.S. Government Printing Office, from Duke University Medical Center Workshop Proceedings, 1972, pp. 177–84.

7. E. M. Brecher and eds., "The 'Heroin Overdose' Mystery and Other Occupational Hazards of Addiction," in: *The Consumer's Union Report: Licit and Illicit Drugs*, Boston: Little, Brown, 1972, pp. 101–14.

8. M. M. Baden, "Medical Aspects of Drug Abuse," *New York Medicine 24:* 1968, pp. 464–68.

9. M. Helpern and Y. Rho, "Deaths from Narcotism in New York City: Incidence, Circumstances and Post-Mortem Findings," *New York State Journal of Medicine 66:* 1966, pp. 2391–408.

10. M. M. Baden, "Investigation of Deaths from Drug Abuse," in: *Mediolegal Investigation of Death: Guidelines for the Application of Pathology to Criminal Investigation*, W. U. Spitz and R. S. Fisher, eds., Springfield, Ill.: Charles C. Thomas, 1973, pp. 485–508.

11. V. P. Dole and M. E. Nyswander, "A Medical Treatment for Diacetylmorphine (Heroin) Addiction: A Clinical Trial with Methadone Hydrochloride," *Journal of American Medical Association 193:* 1965, pp. 646–50; "The Use of Methadone for Narcotic Blockade," *British Journal of Addictions 63:* 1968, pp. 55–57.

12. E. M. Brecher and eds., "Why Methadone Maintenance Works," in: *The Consumers Union Report: Licit and Illicit Drugs*, Boston: Little, Brown, 1972, pp. 159–62.

13. F. R. Gearing, "Methadone Maintenance Treatment Five Years Later— Where Are They Now," *American Journal of Public Health Supplement 64:* 1974, pp. 44–50; F. R. Gearing and M. D. Schweitzer, "An Epidemiological Evaluation of Long-Term Methadone Maintenance Treatment for Heroin Addiction," *American Journal of Epidemiology 100:* 1974, pp. 101–12.

14. A. Richman, G. Jackson, and H. Trigg, "Follow-up of Methadone Maintenance Patients Hospitalized for Abuse of Alcohol and Barbiturates," in: *Fifth National Conference on Methadone Treatment 1973 Proceedings*, R. L. DuPont and R. S. Freeman, eds., New York: NAPAN, 1973, pp. 1484–93.

15. B. Bihari, "Alcoholism in M.M.T.P. Patients: Etiological Factors and Treatment Approaches," see pp. 288–95 in ref. 14.

16. G. J. McKenna et al. "Problems of Mixed Addictions on a Detoxification Unit," see pp. 990–94 in ref. 14.

17. D. R. Wesson, "Acute Treatment of Heroin Addiction with Special Reference to Mixed Drug Addictions: Pt. II: Withdrawal," in: *The Non-Medical Use of Drugs: Contemporary Clinical Issues*, S. Einstein and G. G. DeAngelis, eds., Farmingdale, N. Y.: Behavioral Publishing, 1972, pp. 9–16.

18. Study supported by Contract No. 272761107 from the National Institute on Drug Abuse, Frances Rowe Gearing, principal investigator.

19. G. W. Jackson and A. Richman, "Alcohol Use among Narcotic Addicts," *Alcohol, Health and Research World 1:* 1973, pp. 25–28.

20. M. M. Baden and D. J. Ottenberg, "Alcohol—The All-American Drug of

Choice," L. London, mod., *Contemporary Drug Problems, A Law Quarterly 6:* 1974, pp. 101–125.

21. J. Langrod, "Multiple Drug Use among Heroin Users," in: *Yearbook of Drug Abuse,* L. Brill and E. Harms, eds., New York: Behavioral Publications, 1973, pp. 303–32.

22. C. D. Chambers and M. Moldstead, "The Evolution of Concurrent Opiate and Sedative Addictions," in: *The Epidemiology of Opiate Addiction in the United States,* J. C. Ball and C. D. Chambers, eds., Springfield, Ill.: Charles C. Thomas, 1970, pp. 130–46.

23. Study supported by Grant No. 1-R01-DA-00481 from the National Institute on Drug Abuse, Michael M. Baden, principal investigator, report, December, 1977.

24. *Methadone Treatment Manual,* Washington, D. C.: National Institute of Law Enforcement and Criminal Justice, June 1973, p. 14.

25. R. L. DuPont, Preface, in: L. N. Robins, *The Vietnam Drug User Returns,* Washington, D. C.: Special Action Office for Drug Abuse Prevention, Series A., No. 1, 1974.

26. Statistics from New York State Economic Development Board, 1975 and U.S. Veterans Administration, 1974.

27. P. W. Haberman and M. M. Baden, "Drinking, Drugs and Death," *International Journal of the Addictions 9:* 1974, pp. 761–73.

Photographs Taken During Investigation of Deaths Associated with Substance Abuse

From Office of Chief Medical Examiner, New York City

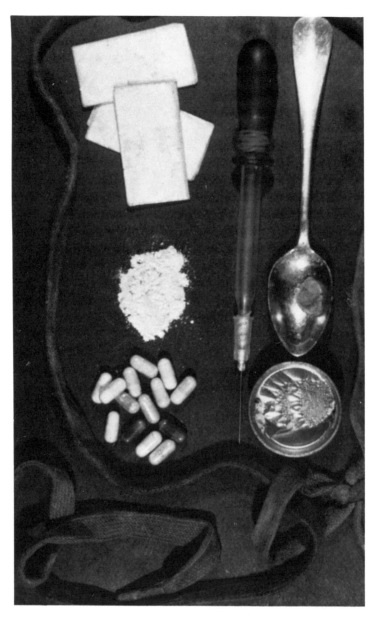

"Works" found at the scene of death of narcotics addict who died of an acute narcotic reaction. Note the homemade eye dropper syringe, bottle-top and spoon containing cotton used as "cooker" to dissolve the narcotic; the packaging of narcotics in a glassine envelope and gelatin capsules; white powder contents of one bag (5% narcotic and 95% diluents); and shoelace tourniquet.

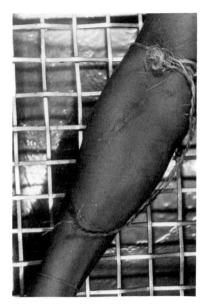

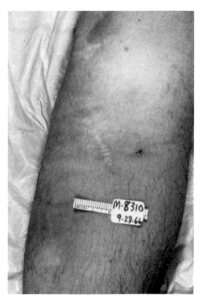

Thirty-three-year-old male, a chronic intravenous heroin addict, died with rope tourniquet still tied around elbow following narcotics injection. Note prominent needle-track scar.

Fresh needle puncture and old pale needle-track scar of 35-year-old male. He was a chronic intravenous heroin addict who died of an acute narcotic reaction soon after injecting the mixture of street heroin.

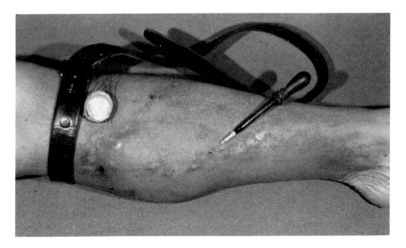

Forty-seven-year-old male narcotics abuser found dead with a needle and syringe still in leg vein. He was using lower extremity veins for injection because his arms were inspected daily for injection sites at MMTP where he was being treated.

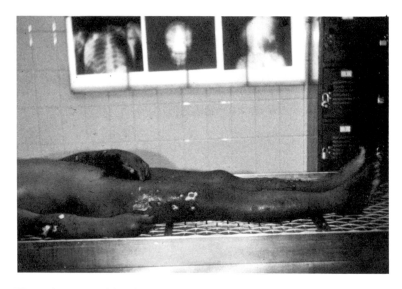

Thirty-three-year-old male "skin popper" (subcutaneous narcotics user) shot during holdup attempt. Note the open and healed abscesses at the injection sites and the swelling of the arms and hands due to venous and lymphatic obstructions by the skin-popping scars.

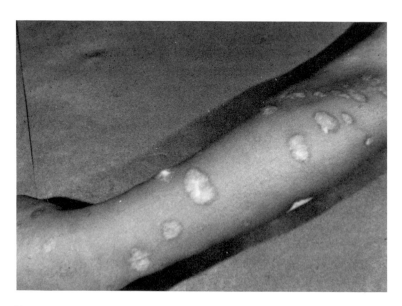

Skin-popping scars of a 39-year-old female heroin addict who died of tetanus.

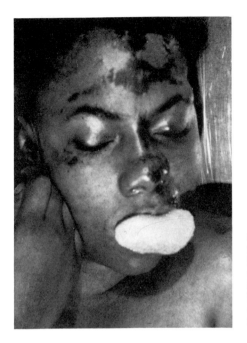

Gray froth exuding from mouth (in shaving cream fashion) of 19-year-old woman following heroin injection. Note postmortem bruising of face due to dragging of the body to a nonincriminating area.

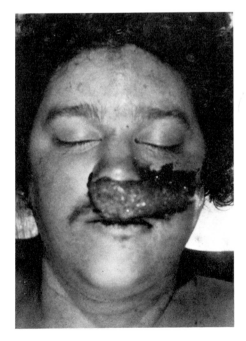

Froth mixed with slight amount of blood exuding from nose of 21-year-old male following illicit use of methadone.

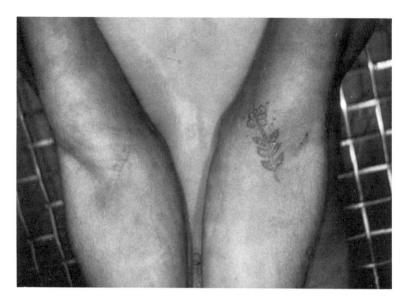

Twenty-three-year-old male attempted to hide needle track scars with a tattoo of a flower. He died following a heroin injection.

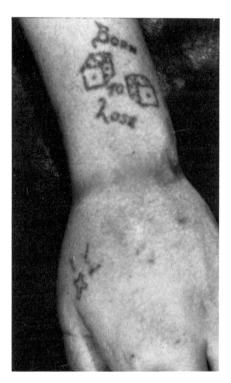

Common tattoos in heroin addicts—"born to lose"; dice showing snake eyes and the antisocial pacheco cross with the three lines above it —on a 23-year-old male who died following a heroin injection. These are "homemade" tattoos, often acquired in jail.

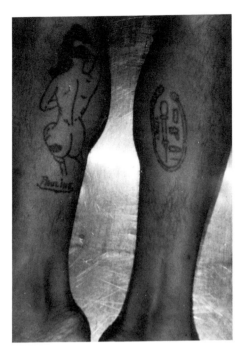

"Works" tattooed on inner aspect of left leg of a 37-year-old male. Tattooing of a needle and syringe invariably means that person is a narcotics addict. He died as a result of gunshot wounds.

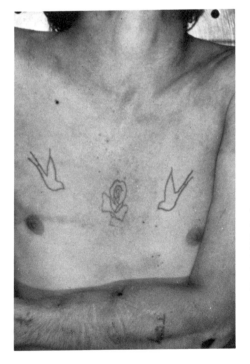

Twenty-six-year-old male with many "homemade, jailhouse-type" tattoos: pacheco on left wrist; "Tony," the decedent's boyfriend; and doves over nipples suggesting homosexuality. Note the abscess at the heroin injection site. He died of acute and chronic intravenous narcotism.

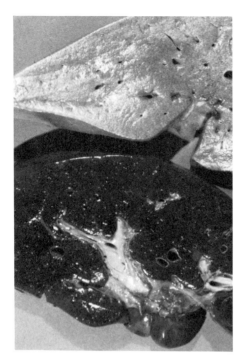

Fatty liver (top), identifiable by its yellowish color, with lobular architecture intact, in a 58-year-old male chronic alcoholic. Note the contrast with a normal maroon-brown liver (below).

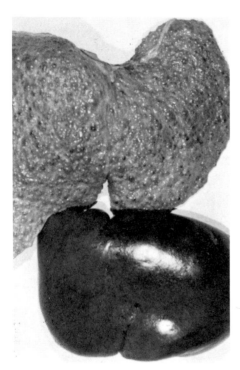

Fatty cirrhotic liver with prominent nodularity in a 45-year-old chronic alcoholic. Note enlarged spleen. He died of bleeding esophageal varices.

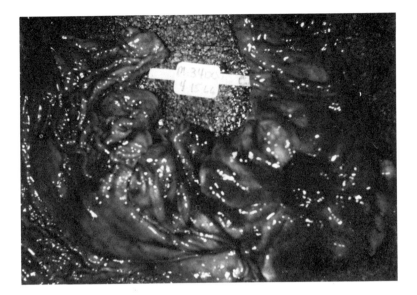

Middle: Natural death in a 50-year-old male alcoholic, resulting from a large, chronic peptic ulcer at beginning of duodenum with penetration through an artery and exsanguination. Ulcers are found more frequently in alcoholics than in nonalcoholics.

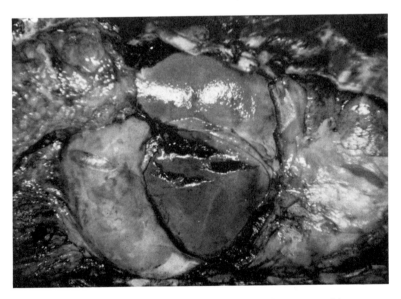

Unnatural death in a 25-year-old male alcoholic, from lacerations of fatty liver seen in situ. Subject was kicked in the abdomen during a homicidal assault.

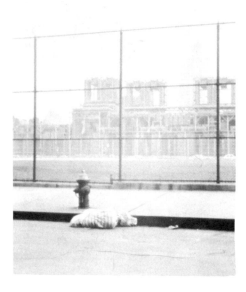

Twenty-four-year-old female heroin addict who died following a heroin injection. Her body was wrapped in the bedspread and dumped. No attempt was made to disguise her identity; personal effects were found with the body.

Alcohol abuse is often linked to homicides; in this case, an intoxicated patron shot a 60-year-old female bartender during a quarrel.

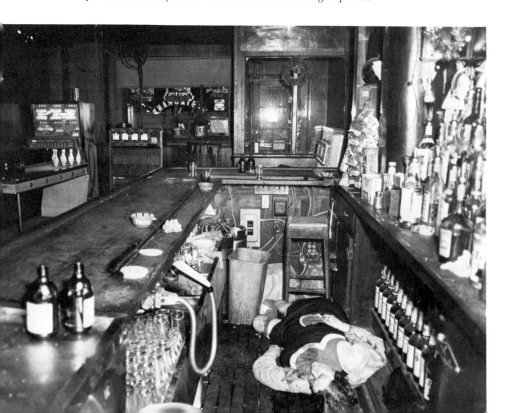

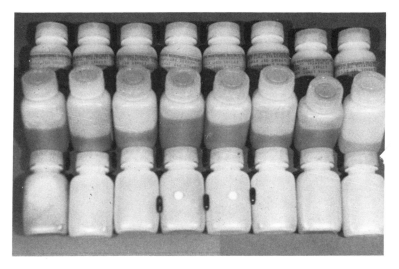

Twenty-four medication bottles containing methadone surreptitiously hoarded by addict in treatment program. Found during investigation of death from acute methadone poisoning after illicit sale.

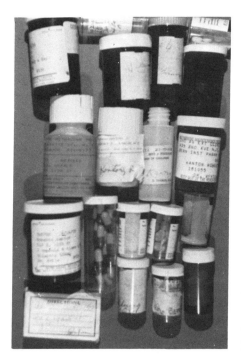

Methadone and tranquilizers given to narcotics abuser enrolled in four different Methadone Maintenance Treatment Programs (MMTP) simultaneously, and taken at a party by two friends who later died of methadone poisoning.

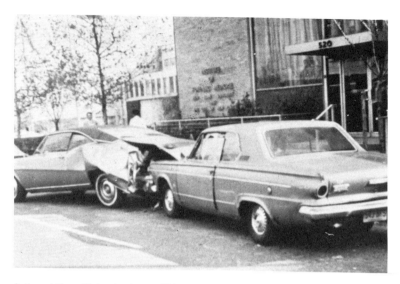

Automobile collision in front of Medical Examiner's Office in New York City. The driver struck another car from behind; his blood alcohol concentration (BAC) was 0.11%.

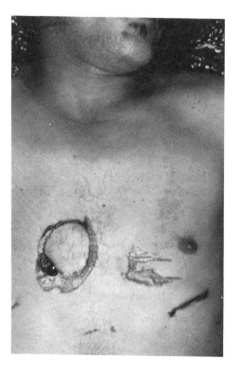

The driver of auto with fatal impact injuries incurred against steering wheel and steering column when his car struck an abutment. The BAC in this 30-year-old male was 0.28%. His ribs were fractured and his heart was lacerated.

5

Suicides, Homicides, and Fatal Accidents

A strong positive association between physical evidence of alcoholism and suicide (1,2), homicide (3), traffic fatalities (4,5), and other fatal accidents (4) has been revealed consistently in the findings of relevant studies. A review of the literature by Blum and Braunstein confirms this link between problem drinking and violent causes of death (6). High blood alcohol concentrations (BACs) have been found in substantial percentages of persons whose deaths were due to suicide (1,7), homicide (1,8), and motor vehicle (9) or other accidents (10). Excessive mortality from all violent causes is also associated with narcotics use (11,12), with homicide being by far the most common (13,14). Alcoholics tend to be more equally distributed than narcotics addicts among all three categories of violent death (6).

Determination of Violent Death Categories

There are two different aspects to a medical examiner's investigation of apparently or possibly unnatural deaths. The first involves the determination of the underlying cause of death which may be a gunshot wound or head trauma, infectious disease such as hepatitis or tetanus, or other diseases such as cirrhosis of the liver or occlusive coronary arteriosclerosis. The second aspect concerns the certification of the mode or manner of death as natural, accident, suicide, or homicide. For example, a fatal injury to the head may occur because of an accidental fall, suicidal jump, or homicidal push; hepatitis may or may not be caused by a dirty needle used by a narcotics addict; and cirrhosis of the liver may or may not be due to alcohol abuse. Our concern in this chapter is with the latter aspect—determining the mode or manner of violent deaths.

A major problem in these investigations is to determine whether violent deaths were accidental or suicidal. An evaluation of the scene and circumstances of the death, history from friends and relatives, examination of the body, and postmortem physical findings may establish or disprove homicide as the mode of death. Certification of suicide depends on an appropriate history from a witness, a suicide note or threats, a previous attempt, a history of mental illness or depression, or a motive (such as a family tragedy, major financial or business reversal, or serious illness); whether or not the acts leading to death are intentional must also be determined.

The final certification as to the mode of death in possible suicide cases often depends on the information provided by the toxicologist, police, or relatives—especially in cases of drug overdose, jumping from heights, hanging, or drowning. In such cases a temporary death certificate is issued to permit burial of the body. The certificate usually includes a phrase such as "pending further study." Sometimes in New York City and in other busy jurisdictions, these cases are backlogged without a certification of "suicide" unless a final determination is requested by relatives or insurance companies. Health departments commonly report these incomplete data which are often utilized by the casual researcher without a review of the files on completed suicidal cases available in medical examiners' offices.

Uniform international mortality statistics have been successfully developed in the World Health Organization's publication of *International Classification of Diseases* (15). According to the seventh revision of that publication, in effect from 1955 to 1968 (16), deaths caused by jumps or falls from heights, ingestion of poison, and inhalation of gas, even when the specific circumstances were not fully determinable, were certified as suicides because the great majority of such deaths, when sufficient evidence was available, proved to be suicidal. However, the mode of deaths due to ingestion of drugs and drowning under such circumstances remained uncertified. According to the eighth revision of the *International Classification of Diseases*, in effect since 1969 (15), all of these causes of death are to be certified as undetermined when suicidal or accidental circumstances cannot be proven — resulting in a spurious decrease in the reported number of suicides.

When the circumstances are not completely determinable, certain specific causes of death are more likely than others to be certified as suicides. For example, if only one non-narcotic drug were taken, the death is more likely to be considered suicidal. On the other hand, if narcotics were used alone or with other drugs, the death is more likely to be considered "narcotism." When there is toxicologic evidence of a narcotic drug, the possibility that substances were taken to produce euphoria usually becomes sufficient to preclude intent to commit suicide. Furthermore, death usually does not result from sublethal amounts of one drug added to sublethal amounts of alcohol or other drugs. There is undoubtedly an underreporting of suicides by drugs in most other areas of the United States because this determination cannot be made without an autopsy and good toxicology. In many jurisdictions, autopsies and toxicologic tests are not performed unless there is sufficient suspicion of suicidal intent.

Adults hit by trains after a fall or jump from a station platform are usually considered suicide victims. The train operator in such cases is very often the only witness and he generally testifies that the victim jumped intentionally rather than fell accidentally, though such testimony may be a rationalization that the operator could not have prevented the death. Without a note or other grounds for suicide, or evidence of sudden natural death, fatal traffic accidents involving only one motor vehicle and occupant are certified as accidental. Some percentage of these accidents, however, are surely suicidal in intent, probably more frequently on rural high-speed highways than in a city like New York.

There is undoubtedly a tendency for relatives to withhold information which would support a certification of suicide because of the social stigma, respect for the deceased, or the risk of losing third-party payments to beneficiaries which is becoming an increasingly important factor. The net effect is an increase in the reported rates for fatal accidents to offset the underreporting of suicides.

In our study, all potential suicide cases including a few that had not yet been certified as to the mode of death were assigned a mode using consistent methods. Once a case was categorized as a homicide, its status in our study remained unchanged even in the event that an alleged perpetrator was not indicted or was found innocent. Likewise, the homicidal intent—whether premeditated, uncalculated, or justifiable—did not affect the status of our homicide cases. However, persons who were unintentionally killed as a result of traffic accidents, including hit-and-run victims, even when there was a charge of criminally negligent homicide or manslaughter were categorized as motor-vehicle accident victims.

Alcoholism, Narcotism, and Violent Death

The leading causes of death for persons in our study classified as alcoholics, narcotics abusers, or both were alcoholism and narcotism (see Chapter 4). Substance abusers also comprise sizable proportions of all violent deaths in our study. Moreover, a considerable percentage of these victims, whether classified as substance abusers or nonabusers had taken alcohol and/or other drugs shortly before their death.

The causes of death for the 812 nonabusers (classified as such in the absence of any evident problem with alcohol or narcotics) were concentrated in the categories of homicides, accidents, and suicides, in that order (Table 5.1, top). Apart from substance abuse, homicide was also the leading cause of death in the other three subgroups, particularly narcotics abusers. Thirty-two percent of the narcotics abusers, 18 percent of the alcoholics, and 18 percent of those with both conditions were homicide victims. In those three subgroups, only the alcoholics had an appreciable proportion of deaths from suicide, motor vehicle accidents (drivers, passengers, or pedestrians), or other accidents (mostly falls, fires, or drownings). Approximately 10 percent of the alcoholics were in each of those cause-of-death categories.

The role of alcohol and narcotics in homicides, suicides, and fatal accidents, however, is somewhat obscured when the totals include the proportion of victims whose deaths were caused directly by ei-

Table 5–1. Cause of Death for Persons Classified as Alcoholics and/or Narcotics Abusers

CAUSE-OF-DEATH CERTIFICATION	N:	ALCOHOLICS (581)	NARCOTICS ABUSERS (339)	BOTH CONDITIONS (222)	NON-ABUSERS (812)
Natural		7.2%	1.8%	0.5%	1.1%
Accident					
Motor vehicle		7.9	1.8	0.9	18.5
Other		8.8	2.9	4.5	13.7
Suicide		10.5	7.1	4.5	29.7
Homicide		18.2	31.6	17.6	36.2
Alcoholism[a]		47.0	n.a.*	16.7	n.a.
Narcotism[a]		n.a.	54.6	27.9	n.a.
Alcoholism and					
narcotism		n.a.	n.a.	27.0	n.a.
Other drug(s)					
poisoning		0.3	0.3	0.5	0.9
Total		100%	100%	100%	100%

Classification of Persons as Alcoholics and/or Narcotics Abusers According to Cause of Death

CAUSE-OF-DEATH CERTIFICATION	N	ALCO-HOLICS	NARCOTICS ABUSERS	BOTH CONDI-TIONS	NON-ABUSERS	TOTAL
Natural	(58)	72.4%	10.3	1.7	15.5	100%
Accident						
Motor vehicle	(204)	22.5	2.9	1.0	73.5	100
Other	(182)	28.0	5.5	5.5	61.0	100
Suicide	(336)	18.2	7.1	3.0	71.7	100
Homicide	(546)	19.4	19.6	7.1	53.8	100
Alcoholism[a]	(310)	88.1	n.a.	11.9	n.a.	100
Narcotism[a]	(247)	n.a.	74.9	25.1	n.a.	100
Alcoholism and						
narcotism	(60)	n.a.	n.a.	100.0	n.a.	100
Other drug(s)						
poisoning	(11)	18.2	9.1	9.1	63.6	100

a. Alcoholism and/or narcotism alone or with other cause of death.

*n.a. = not applicable.

ther or both of these substances. To give a clearer picture, alcoholics, narcotics abusers, and those with both conditions are shown as a proportion of all homicide, suicide, and accident victims at the bottom of Table 5.1. Of the 546 adult homicide victims, 46 percent were classified as substance abusers. Similarly, 29 percent of all suicides,

Table 5–2. BAC and Other Toxicology for Suicide, Homicide, and Accident Victims

| CAUSE OF DEATH | BLOOD OR BRAIN ALCOHOL CONCENTRATION (BAC) | | | |
	N^a	*Negative*	*.01 – .09%*	*.10% or above*	*Total*
Suicide					
Ingestion of pills	(90)	65.6%	18.9	15.6	100%
Other	(157)	70.1%	13.4	16.6	100%
Sum	(247)	68.4%	15.4	16.2	100%
Homicide	(499)	58.1%	15.2	26.7	100%
Motor vehicle accident					
Driver	(61)	47.5%	14.8	37.7	100%
Passenger	(25)	76.0%	8.0	16.0	100%
Pedestrian[b]	(61)	70.5%	8.2	21.3	100%
Sum	(147)	61.9%	10.9	27.2	100%
Other accident					
Fall	(54)	51.9%	7.4	40.7	100%
Fire	(28)	46.4%	7.1	46.4	100%
Drowning	(19)	42.1%	15.8	52.6	100%
Sum[c]	(121)	47.1%	9.9	43.0	100%

a. Total N and proportions with BAC and other toxicology obtained:

	N	BAC	other toxicology
Suicide			
Ingestion of pills	(96)	93.8%	94.8%
Other	(240)	65.4	65.4
Homicide	(546)	91.4	91.2
Motor vehicle accident			
Driver	(74)	82.4	82.4
Passenger	(33)	75.8	75.8
Pedestrian	(97)	62.9	62.9
Other accident	(182)	66.5	65.9

b. Includes total of 10 hit-and-run cases.

28 percent of all motor vehicle fatalities, and 39 percent of other accident victims were alcoholics, narcotics abusers, or both. Alcoholics, in particular, contributed large proportions to each of these violent death categories—ranging from 18 percent of the suicides to 28 percent of the other accident victims.

According to discussions with the police and district attorneys, many perpetrators of homicides are narcotics addicts or are intoxicated when committing the murder so that well over one-half of all homicides of adults in New York City may involve substance abusers

Table 5-2. Continued

CAUSE OF DEATH		OTHER TOXICOLOGY[d]			
				Other mood-altering drugs	
	N^a	Negative	Narcotics	only	Total
Suicide					
Ingestion of pills	(91)	6.6%	6.6	86.8	100%
Other	(157)	70.1%	7.6	22.3	100%
Sum	(248)	47.2%	7.3	45.6	100%
Homicide	(498)	76.9%	17.7	5.4	100%
Motor vehicle accident					
Driver	(61)	88.5%	1.6	9.8	100%
Passenger	(25)	80.0%	12.0	8.0	100%
Pedestrian[b]	(61)	86.9%	3.3	9.8	100%
Sum	(147)	86.4%	4.1	9.5	100%
Other accident					
Fall	(53)	79.2%	9.4	11.3	100%
Fire	(27)	77.8%	3.7	18.5	100%
Drowning	(19)	94.7%	—	5.3	100%
Sum[c]	(120)	83.3%	5.8	10.8	100%

c. Includes total of 25 other accidents.
d. Toxicology categories for drugs other than alcohol:
   Negative—no mood-altering drugs present.
   Narcotics—morphine (heroin metabolite) or methadone with or without other mood-altering drug(s).
   Other mood-altering drugs only—primarily hypnotics (mostly barbiturates) and tranquilizers.

as either victims, perpetrators, or both. Alcohol is also implicated in many other violent deaths of nonabusers, such as pedestrians struck by drunk drivers and persons who die in fires resulting from the carelessness of someone who is drunk. It is very difficult to estimate how often alcohol or other drugs influence the perpetrator of a homicide or survivor at fault in an accidental death because the living are not subject to the same immediate toxicologic testing as the dead, for legal or temporal reasons.

It has been observed that about one-half of all violent deaths are associated with alcohol use (17). Moreover, an approximately equal amount of alcohol use has been reported to occur among the offenders in cases of homicide and other fatal violence (8,18). When medical examiner cases involving narcotic users are added to these, the totals indicate more than two-thirds of the violent deaths in New York City are associated with the use or abuse of these substances by the victims, perpetrators, or both.

Alcohol and Drug Use before Violent Death

The BAC and other toxicologic results for the suicide, homicide, and accident victims in our sample (see Table 5.2, p. 80–81) reveal the importance of alcohol and other mood-altering drugs as a precipitating factor in these violent deaths. The dangers of driving while under the influence of alcohol have been well publicized. Some lesser known relationships between alcohol or other drugs and violent deaths are also demonstrated by these data.

In all categories except suicide, the alcohol levels were likely to be 0.10 percent or more for victims with positive BACs. About three drinks of whiskey (4 1/2 ounces) or the equivalent must be consumed in one hour to reach this alcohol level, which usually results in impairment or intoxication. Even more often than motor vehicle drivers, those who died from fires, falls, or drownings had BACs of 0.10 percent or more at the time of death. Many pedestrians hit by motor vehicles (as well as passengers) in our sample also showed postmortem evidence of alcohol. Although a BAC of 0.10 percent is legally considered evidence in New York of driving while intoxicated, many persons will be impaired at lower blood alcohol levels. We fully agree with Larson's recommendation that all persons be forbidden by law to drive with a BAC of more that 0.05 percent (19).

More than one-half of the fatally injured motor vehicle drivers and other accident victims had positive BACs. The proportion with alcohol levels of 0.10 percent or more ranged from 38 percent of the drivers to 53 percent of the drowning victims. Alcohol has also been found to be a factor in a large percentage of drownings in jurisdictions other than New York City. A BAC greater than 0.10 percent was found in about one-third of the victims by coroners and medical examiners in various U.S. cities and states in 1974 (20). Forty-two percent of the homicide victims had some alcohol in their system and 27 percent had levels of at least 0.10 percent. The comparable percentages for suicide, pedestrian, and passenger fatalities were somewhat smaller, except for 15 percent of suicide victims with BACs of .01 to .09 percent, suggesting that many suicide victims had a drink or two, perhaps to release inhibitions, before taking their lives.

Except for persons who committed suicide by taking an overdose of pills, alcohol was used more than any other mood-altering substance by a larger percentage of victims in all cause-of-death categories. Barbiturates, other sedatives, hypnotics, and/or tranquilizers were detected in 86 percent of the toxicologic examinations of suicide victims who had taken an overdose of pills. In a small percentage of these suicide cases, Darvon (propoxyphene) (13%) and narcotics (7%) were also found alone or in conjunction with other drugs. Nonnarcotic drugs—mostly tranquilizers and barbiturates—were detected in toxicologic tests on 22 percent of the suicide victims from other causes, 18 percent of the fire victims, and on about 10 percent of the other fatalities. Narcotics were most often present in homicide victims, 18 percent having toxicologic evidence of recent heroin and/or methadone use.

Demographic Characteristics of Victims

Demographic similarities and differences between substance abusers and nonabusers in the four violent death categories are presented in Table 5.3. Narcotics abusers who have also been classified as alcoholics are combined with those classified as only narcotics abusers here because of their demographic comparability which was discussed in Chapter 4. These findings may be interpreted according to either (a) the classification of decedents as alcoholics, narcotics abusers, and nonabusers or (b) their cause of death.

More of the 336 suicide victims than those in other violent death categories, irrespective of their classification as alcoholics, narcotics abusers, or nonabusers, were women and white (38% and 62%, respectively), and a relatively large percentage were reported to be sick most of the year before their death. As indicated by the medical examiners and our interviewers, most of the 23 percent reported to be sick had symptoms of depression or other mental illness. Homicide victims most often were poorly educated, Hispanic or black men, regardless of their classification as substance abusers or nonabusers.

Table 5–3. Selected Demographic Characteristics of Alcoholics, Narcotics Abusers, and Nonabusers in Violent Death Categories

SELECTED CHARACTERISTICS		PERCENTAGES ACCORDING TO CAUSE OF DEATH			
		Suicide	*Homicide*	*Motor Vehicle Accident*	*Other Accident*
	N:	(61)	(106)	(46)	(51)
Alcoholics					
Male		68.9%	88.7%	82.6%	84.3%
Median age		46 yrs.	45 yrs.	46 yrs.	47 yrs.
High school graduate or more		42.7%	24.5%	34.8%	39.3%
Ethnicity[a]					
Hispanic[b]		14.8%	34.3%	30.4%	21.6%
Black		24.6	40.0	28.3	35.3
White		60.7	25.7	41.3	43.1
Total		100%	100%	100%	100%
Principal activity in past year					
Sick		26.2%	17.0%	6.5%	21.6%
Substance abuse, nothing, jail		8.2%	9.4%	4.4%	17.6%
Narcotics abusers[c]	N:	(34)	(146)	(8)[d]	(20)
Male		64.7%	90.4%	—	85.0%
Median age		28 yrs.	28 yrs.	—	33 yrs.
High school graduate or more		41.1%	38.3%	—	50.0%
Ethnicity[a]					
Hispanic[b]		20.6%	37.0%	—	30.0%
Black		26.5	52.1	—	50.0
White		52.9	11.0	—	20.0
Total		100%	100%	—	100%
Principal activity in past year					
Sick		14.7%	4.8%	—	30.0%
Substance abuse, nothing, jail		26.5%	28.8%	—	25.0
Nonabusers	N:	(241)	(294)	(150)	(111)
Male		60.6%	69.6%	67.3%	73.0%
Median age		37 yrs.	34 yrs.	52 yrs.	46 yrs.
High school graduate or more		68.5%	40.2%	50.0%	46.8%
Ethnicity[a]					
Hispanic[b]		14.1%	28.9%	16.2%	20.0%
Black		20.1	42.6	12.8	35.5
White		65.8	28.5	70.9	44.5
Total		100%	100%	100%	100%
Principal activity in past year					
Sick		23.2%	5.1%	7.3%	16.2%
Substance abuse, nothing, jail		4.1%	5.5%	2.0%	5.4%

Of the 546 homicide victims, 84 percent were men, 76 percent were Hispanics or blacks, and 53 percent were not high school graduates. The characteristics of all homicide and suicide cases in our study, whether they were classified as substance abusers or nonabusers, confirm previous findings that in the United States homicide victims are predominantly nonwhite, lower-class males. Although the majority of suicide victims are also males, a somewhat larger proportion are white females (8,21,22).

Although the alcoholics were much older than the narcotics abusers, their ages did not vary much according to the causes of death (Table 5.3). The median age for alcoholics was 45 to 47 years and for narcotics abusers, 28 to 33 years. Among the nonabusers, the homicide and suicide victims tended to be younger than the accident fatalities. The median ages for nonabusers who were homicide, suicide, traffic, or other accident victims were 34, 37, 52, and 46 years, respectively. Many of the persons who died as a result of nontraffic accidents, whether or not they were substance abusers, were reported to be sick or engaged in nonproductive activities—substance abuse, nothing, or jail—most of the year before they died. Nineteen percent of the 182 other accident victims were reported to be sick, and 11 percent were doing nothing productive most of the previous year.

The motor-vehicle accident victims in our study include drivers, pedestrians, and passengers, three groups with very different demographic characteristics. The 74 drivers were almost all men (95%), and 46 percent were less than 30 years old. The 97 pedestrians were mostly men (65%) who were older than the drivers, 71 percent being 50 years of age or more. Most of the 33 passengers were women (61%) and 42 percent were in the 18–29 age group. Overall, 63 percent of

Table 5–3 (notes)

a. Excludes one Oriental homicide.

b. Decedent or at least one parent born in Puerto Rico or Spanish-speaking country in Western Hemisphere, irrespective of color.

c. Includes 61 (29.3%) who were classified as both narcotics abusers and alcoholics.

d. *N* too small for percentages.

e. Excludes seven suicides, three homicides, two motor vehicle accident victims, and one other accident victim who were Orientals.

the motor vehicle fatalities were white, and there was little difference in ethnicity among the three groups of traffic victims. These sex and age distributions of fatally injured drivers and pedestrians in our study are comparable to national statistics for the same time period (20) and data from other studies done in urban areas (5). As in our study, pedestrians usually outnumbered drivers in mortality data from other urban areas (5,20).

Alcoholism has been described as a form of "chronic suicide" and a manifestation of self-destructive tendencies by Menninger (23); others have viewed it as a substitute for a more rapidly lethal means of self-destruction (24), or a suicidal equivalent. Indeed, 263 persons in our study died of chronic alcoholism alone or with another cause excluding narcotism. In addition, 61 persons classified as alcoholics committed suicide. Those who died of alcoholism, in a manner of speaking, let the disease run its course, whereas the others abruptly terminated the process by taking their own lives. In our study, these two groups were in some respects very similar and in others, rather different. They had almost the same median age, comparable sex ratios, and equivalent educational attainment. The median age was 47 for those who died of alcoholism and 46 for the alcoholic suicide victims; 75 percent and 69 percent, respectively, were men; and 43 percent in both groups were high school graduates or more highly educated. Comparably large proportions, 25 percent of the alcoholism decedents and 26 percent of the suicide victims, were reported to be sick most of the year preceding their death. Our impressions were that almost all of those who died of alcoholism suffered from chronic symptoms of the disease, whereas most of the alcoholic suicide victims had manifest signs of mental illness, most commonly, depression.

There were marked differences between these groups of alcoholics in ethnicity and marital status. Larger proportions of those who died of alcoholism were blacks, most of whom were born in the South, and more who had never been married. The suicide victims were predominantly white, and twice as many were married at the time of death. For their principal activity in the past year before death, more of the alcoholics who committed suicide were reported to be in the labor force, while more of those who died of alcoholism were reported to be drinking or doing nothing. These percentages for the two groups are:

	CAUSE OF DEATH:	CHRONIC ALCOHOLISM	SUICIDE
	N:	(263)	(61)
Ethnicity			
Black		44.1%	24.6%
White		43.7	60.7
Marital status			
Never married		31.6	21.3
Married at time of death		22.1	41.0
Principal activity in past year			
Working, looking for work, laid off (in labor force)		28.9	37.7
Drinking or nothing		18.3	8.2

In studies of suicide and alcoholism, suicide rates have been consistently lower among blacks than among whites (1). One hypothesis to account for the lower rates of suicide among black alcoholics is that attitudes toward heavy drinking may be more permissive among blacks than among whites in comparable socioeconomic groups, and heavy drinking may be a larger part of the overall life patterns of the lower-class blacks (25).

Our data indicate that if alcoholics are white, married, and in the labor force, they are more likely to commit suicide. We can speculate that they more frequently had spouses, other relatives, and employers who objected to their drinking. Conversely, black alcoholics who were single and whose principal activity seemed to be drinking or doing nothing died of chronic alcoholism more often, perhaps indicating an absence of conflict over their drinking and its consequences.

Most of the 247 narcotism deaths in our study were primarily due to an acute reaction; only 24 suicide victims were classified as solely narcotics abusers. Therefore, our comparison between alcoholics who died of chronic alcoholism or committed suicide could not be repeated with the narcotics abusers.

Victims and Perpetrators

A list of all motor vehicle operators charged with driving while intoxicated who had survived fatal traffic accidents during the twelve-month period when our informants were being interviewed was prepared by the Aided and Accident Section of the New York City Police Department. Twenty-one intoxicated drivers were involved in fatal accidents that had occurred in the Bronx, Manhattan, Queens, or Staten Island and were thus investigated at the Chief Medical Examiner's Office in Manhattan. Six of these drivers charged with driving while intoxicated were involved with motor vehicle fatalities in our sample. Approximately 120 drivers survived fatal traffic accidents in our study, so that the six who were identified as being intoxicated provide some fragmentary evidence of the consequences of alcohol abuse on innocent victims.

Relationships between homicide victims and perpetrators and the homicide motives were examined with the help of the Crime Analysis Section of the New York City Police Department in March of 1976. The most recent Police Department information on the criminal histories of our cases up to the time of indictment or trial was tabulated in preparing Table 5.4. In earlier reports on this subject by Wolfgang and others, the great majority of murderers have been relatives, friends, or acquaintances of the victims. The motive most often has been a dispute, and almost 90 percent of homicides were resolved (8,21). Most studies on homicide perpetrators, however, extrapolate from the resolved cases which are greatly skewed toward those committed by relatives or friends. In the past decade, with drug addiction becoming a much more important factor in homicides in New York City, a much larger number are committed by nonrelatives, and these are less often resolved. Thus at present less than 60 percent of the homicides in New York City are resolved (26).

Thirty-nine percent of the perpetrators of the 546 homicides in our study were friends or acquaintances of the victims and 8 percent were relatives. The motive was a dispute in 46 percent of our cases. Strangers committed 27 percent of the homicides, and the motive in 21 percent was a crime such as robbery. It should be noted, however, that the relationship in 23 percent, and the motive in 17 percent of the cases were still unknown in March of 1976.

Table 5–4. Relationship between Homicide Victims and Perpetrators, and Motives for Homicide According to Classification as Alcoholics, Narcotics Abusers, or Nonabusers

RELATIONSHIP AND MOTIVE		CLASSIFICATION OF VICTIMS			
			Narcotics	*Non-*	
		Alcoholics	*Abusers*[a]	*abusers*	*Sum*
	N:	(106)	(146)	(294)	(546)
Perpetrator's relation-ship to victim					
Relative		12.3%	3.4%	9.5%	8.4%[b]
Friend or acquaintance		29.2	47.3	37.8	38.6
Stranger		31.1	19.9	29.3	27.1
Police		2.8	4.1	2.4	2.9
Unknown		24.5	25.3	21.1	22.9
Total		100%	100%	100%	100%
Motive for homicide					
Dispute		49.1%	45.9%	44.6%	45.7%
Crime, e.g., robbery		22.6	14.4	24.5	21.4
Narcotics		1.8	13.0	5.8	7.0
Other		8.5	7.5	10.5	9.2[c]
Unknown		17.9	19.2	14.6	16.6
Total		100%	100%	100%	100%

a. Includes 39 (26.7%) who were classified as both narcotics abusers and alcoholics.

b. Includes 2.7% legal marriages and 2.6% common-law marriages.

c. Includes 1.3% sex, 0.7% organized crime, 0.5% youth gang, and 6.7% unspecified.

There are a few noteworthy differences among our homicide cases according to whether the victims were alcoholics, narcotics abusers with or without alcoholism, or nonabusers. Narcotics abusers were most often killed by friends or acquaintances (47%), and least often by relatives (3%) or strangers (20%), suggesting particular risks inherent in the drug culture in which such addicts live. The motive for the murder of narcotics abusers was, as expected, more likely to be labeled "narcotics" (13%), and compared to motives for murder of nonabusers and alcoholics, less likely to be a robbery or other such crime (14%). "Narcotics" was also the motive for the murder of smaller percentages of nonabusers (6%) and alcoholics (2%). The victim—perpetrator relationships and motives among alcoholics and nonabusers were comparable, although a relatively larger proportion of nonabusers (38%) than alcoholics (29%) were killed by friends or acquaintances.

The most common means of committing suicide used by the 336 victims in our study were jumping from heights (32%), and taking an overdose of pills (29%); followed by shooting (13%), hanging (8%), and jumping in front of subways (5%). These statistics differ slightly from the overall proportions in New York City, which show pills to be the most common means of suicide, particularly among women, whites, and older persons—followed by jumping, especially by men, blacks, and younger persons. The alcoholics and narcotics abusers in our study who committed suicide were somewhat more likely to use pills, whereas nonabusers tended to jump from heights more often.

Despite the strict gun control laws which severely limit the possession, concealment, and use of handguns, rifles, and shotguns in New York City (27), 53 percent of the 546 homicide victims in our study were killed with guns, excluding 4 percent killed while committing a crime. Of the remainder, 26 percent died of stab wounds, 15 percent of assault, and 4 percent by some other means. Guns were more commonly used as the weapon in deaths of narcotics abusers and nonabusers, whereas alcoholics tended to die more often from stab wounds or assault.

Firearms are used in about two-thirds of all homicides and in one-half of all suicides in the United States, which is only about 15 percent more often as a murder weapon but almost 40 percent more often as a suicide weapon than in New York City (28). Perhaps due to the strict gun control laws in New York City, potential suicide victims may be much less likely than murderers to have legal or illegal guns in their possession, and the means utilized to commit suicide in general conform to the availability of such means. Many more persons commit suicide in New York City by jumping from heights, undoubtedly because of the accessibility of tall buildings. There were about 1.2 suicides for every homicide in the United States in 1974 (28), while in New York City, as reflected in our sample, there were only 0.6 suicides for every homicide.

Summary

Although substance abuse was the major cause of death of persons classified as alcoholics, narcotics abusers, and those with both conditions, many died of violent causes. Homicide was the most frequent violent cause among substance abusers, particularly narcotics abusers. Homicide, accident, and suicide, in that order, were the leading causes of death for nonabusers. Alcohol, more than any other drug, was present in postmortem chemical tests. A majority of the drowning, fire, and motor-vehicle driver victims had positive BACs, with substantial percentages having levels of 0.10 percent or more. Large percentages of other violent death victims also had alcohol present. Narcotics was detected most frequently in homicide victims; other mood-altering drugs were present most often in suicide victims. Demographic characteristics of victims varied according to: (a) their classification as alcoholics, narcotics abusers or nonabusers, and (b) their violent death category. Almost half of the homicide victims in our study knew the perpetrators, and the motive for about the same percentage was a dispute. Jumping from heights and taking an overdose of pills were the most common means of committing suicide; guns were the murder weapons in more than half of our homicide cases. In contrast to national statistics, homicides occurred more often than suicides in our New York City sample.

References

1. D. W. Goodwin, "Alcohol in Homicide and Suicide," *Quarterly Journal of Studies on Alcohol 34:* 1973, pp. 144–56.
2. W. A. Rushing, "Alcoholism and Suicide Rates by Status Set and Occupation," *Quarterly Journal of Studies on Alcohol 29:* 1968, pp. 399–412.
3. S. Y. Choi, "Death in Young Alcoholics," *Journal of Studies on Alcohol 36:* 1975, pp. 1224–29.
4. B. Brenner, "Alcoholism and Fatal Accidents," *Quarterly Journal of Studies on Alcohol 28:* 1967, pp. 517–28.
5. J. A. Waller and H. W. Turkel, "Alcoholism and Traffic Deaths," *New England Journal of Medicine 275:* September 1966, pp. 532–36.
6. R. H. Blum and L. Braunstein, "Mind-Altering Drugs and Dangerous Behavior: Alcohol," in: President's Commission on Law Enforcement and Administration of Justice, *Task Force Report: Drunkenness,* Washington, D.C.: U.S. Government Printing Office, 1967, pp. 29–49.
7. I. P. James, "Blood Alcohol Levels following Successful Suicide," *Quarterly Journal of Studies on Alcohol 27:* 1966, pp. 23–29.
8. M. E. Wolfgang, in: *Studies of Homicide,* M. E. Wolfgang, ed., New York: Harper and Row, 1967, pp. 3–28 and 72–87.
9. M. M. Hyman, "Accident Vulnerability and Blood Alcohol Concentra-

tion of Drivers by Demographic Characteristics," *Quarterly Journal of Studies on Alcohol*, Suppl. No. 4, 1968, pp. 34–57.

10. Metropolitan Life Insurance Co., "Alcohol and Home Accidents at the Working Ages," *Statistical Bulletin 48:* October 1967, pp. 2–4.

11. M. M. Baden, "Homicide, Suicide and Accidental Deaths among Narcotic Addicts," *Human Pathology 3:* 1972, pp. 91–95.

12. G. Vaillant, "A Twelve-Year Follow-Up of New York Narcotic Addicts: Relation of Treatment to Outcome," *American Journal of Psychiatry 122:* 1966, pp. 727–37.

13. E. H. Johnston, L. R. Goldbaum, and R. L. Whelton, "Investigation of Sudden Deaths in Addicts," *Medical Annual, District of Columbia 38:* 1969, pp. 375–80.

14. R. M. Mandel, "A Study of Homicide among Narcotic Users," unpublished report (M. M. Baden, preceptor) *Health Research Training Program, New York City Department of Health,* 1971.

15. National Center for Health Statistics, *International Classification of Diseases, Adapted for Use in the U.S., Eighth Revision,* Washington, D.C.: Public Health Service Publication, 1968, p. 1693.

16. National Center for Health Statistics, *International Classification of Diseases, Adapted for Indexing Hospital Records by Diseases and Operations, Seventh Revision,* Washington, D.C.: Public Health Service Publication 1962, p. 719.

17. M. M. Baden and D. J. Ottenberg, "Alcohol—The All-American Drug of Choice," L. London, mod., *Contemporary Drug Problems, A Law Quarterly 6:* 1974, pp. 101–25.

18. J. Luke, *Office of the Chief Medical Examiner: Annual Report, 1973,* Washington, D. C.: Department of Human Resources, 1973.

19. C. P. Larson, "Alcohol: Fact and Fallacy," in: *Legal Medicine Annual, 1969,* C. H. Wecht, ed., New York: Appleton-Century-Crofts, 1969, pp. 239–68.

20. *Accident Facts, 1976 Edition,* Chicago: National Safety Council, 1976.

21. A. P. Iskrant and P. V. Joliet, *Accidents and Homicide,* Cambridge: Harvard University Press, 1968, pp. 114–21.

22. A. F. Henry and J. F. Short, *Suicide and Homicide,* New York: The Free Press, 1954, pp. 131–40.

23. K. A. Menninger, *Man Against Himself,* New York: Harcourt, Brace, 1938, pp. 160–84.

24. E. G. Palola, T. C. Dorpat, and W. R. Larson, "Alcoholism and Suicidal Behavior," in: *Society, Culture and Drinking Patterns,* D. J. Pittman and C. R. Snyder, eds., New York: Wiley, 1962, pp. 511–34.

25. W. A. Rushing, "Suicide and the Interaction of Alcoholism (Liver Cirrhosis) with the Social Situation," *Quarterly Journal of Studies on Alcohol 30:* 1969, pp. 93–103.

26. S. Raab in *New York Times,* April 20, 1977, pp. A1 and B10.

27. *New York State Penal Law*, Chapter 791, Section 49, Article 400, "Licensing and Other Provisions Relating to Firearms," Laws of New York, 1967, pp. 280–86; *Administrative Code of City of New York*, Police Department, Article 436-5.0, "Firearms," Local Law No. 48, 1964, pp. 814–19.

28. *The CBS News Almanac, 1977*, (Source: U.S. Public Health Service), Maplewood, N.J.: Hammond Almanac, 1976, p. 249.

6

Familial Drinking and Drug-Use Problems

If a disease or condition occurs more often among relatives of persons with the same condition than among comparable nonrelatives, it can be described as familial, with an environmental and/or hereditary etiology. In order to determine whether or not a disease is familial, it is necessary to know its prevalence among relatives of those who have the disease and among nonrelatives drawn from the same population, using equivalent definitions of the disease for the subjects, their relatives, and the nonrelatives.

Before 1960, alcoholism prevalence rates were estimated primarily by the Jellinek formula (1). The formula expressed algebraically is:

$$A = \left(\frac{PD}{K}\right)R \text{ with:}$$

A = the total number of alcoholics alive in a given year
D = the number of reported deaths from liver cirrhosis in that year
P = the percentage of such deaths attributable to alcoholism
K = the percentage of all alcoholics with complications from chronic alcoholism who die of liver cirrhosis
R = the ratio of all alcoholics to alcoholics with complications

Jellinek analyzed trends in mortality from cirrhosis of the liver in relation to periods of prohibition and concluded that there was a sufficiently constant relationship between alcohol consumption and liver cirrhosis mortality to develop a formula for estimating the number of alcoholics in large communities. The formula may have produced reasonable estimates of alcoholism prevalence in the United States for the first decade or so after repeal of Prohibition in 1933. However, each of the three basic constants in the formula, P, K, and R, have undergone numerous changes, so that the formula has been strongly criticized recently as no longer applicable for current estimates. Thus population surveys have been used instead to measure the prevalence of alcoholism in large communities (2).

Two major population surveys were conducted in New York City in the 1960s from which estimated rates of alcoholism or problem drinking were computed. In 1960–61, 2 percent of the adult residents of the Washington Heights Health District in New York City were reported to be probable alcoholics (2), but evidence of a serious underestimate of prevalence was found (3). In a household survey using different methods, 6 percent of adults living in New York City in 1963 were classified as "implicative drinkers" (4). In three nationwide surveys, roughly 7 percent of all adults (10% of all drinkers) have been described as "heavy 'escape' drinkers" by Cahalan (5), "deviant drinkers" by Mulford (6), or compulsive drinkers who probably have difficulties in functioning socially by the National Commission on Marijuana and Drug Abuse (7). Despite the considerable denial of drinking problems by self-respondents and informants and the absence of a precise definition of alcoholism, 7 percent seems a reasonable prevalence rate of alcoholism among adults in the United States (and in New York City). To be classified as a familial disease, the rate of alcoholism among close relatives of alcoholics must be considerably higher than 7 percent—perhaps at least two to three times higher.

The prevalence of problems due to the use of an illicit drug such as heroin may be even more difficult to estimate from population surveys than alcoholism rates because of concealment and denial of illegal activities. A much larger proportion of narcotics users than drinkers, however, have related problems. According to a survey reported in 1976, there were an estimated 230,000 narcotics addicts in New York State, of whom perhaps 90,000 eighteen years of age or older were New York City residents living in the Bronx, Manhattan,

Queens, or Staten Island (8). The population eighteen years of age or older living in these four boroughs of New York City, excluding Brooklyn, was about 3,900,000 (9), so that the overall prevalence rate of narcotics abuse among the adult residents can be estimated at roughly 2 percent.

Familial Rates

If alcoholism and narcotism were familial conditions, the percentage of close relatives — parents, siblings, spouses, or children — reported to have comparable problems should be much greater than 7 percent for alcoholics, and 2 percent for narcotics abusers. As shown in Table 6.1, 15 percent of the alcoholics in our study had one or more close relatives reported to have an alcohol problem, and 9 percent of the

Table 6 – 1. Alcohol and Narcotics Problems Among Close Relatives of Decedents[a]

SUBSTANCE ABUSE BY ONE OR MORE CLOSE RELATIVES		CLASSIFICATION OF DECEDENTS			
		Alcoholics	*Narcotics Abusers*	*Both Conditions*	*Nonabusers*
	N:	(581)	(339)	(222)	(812)
Substance					
Alcohol		14.8%	6.2%	12.6%	2.1%
Narcotics		1.4	9.1	10.4	2.0
Other drugs		0.2	—	0.5	—
None		84.7	85.8	80.6	95.9
Total[b]		101%	101%	104%	100%
Relationship					
Father		7.6%	3.5%	4.1%	1.0%
Mother		2.6	2.1	3.2	0.6
One or more siblings		9.0	9.7	15.3	2.3
Spouse		0.7	0.3	0.9	0.4
Child		0.5	—	—	—
None		84.7	85.8	80.6	95.9
Total[c]		105%	101%	104%	100%

a. Close relatives are parents, siblings, spouse, and children.

b. Totals are greater than 100% because of abuse of more than one substance in some cases.

c. Totals are greater than 100% because more than one close relative was substance abuser in some cases.

narcotics abusers had a relative with a narcotics problem. For those with both conditions, the percentages of close relatives with reported problems were 13 percent for alcohol and 10 percent for narcotics. Thus our familial rates of alcoholism and narcotism based on informants' reports are, respectively, about two and five times the estimated prevalence rates.

Alcohol or other drug problems of close relatives were reported much more often by informants who acknowledged that the decedents had such problems than by those who denied the decedents' problems. Decedents who were classified as alcoholics or narcotics abusers by informants were three times more likely to have close relatives reported to be substance abusers (21%) than alcoholics or narcotics abusers classified by physical evidence alone (7%), as indicated in Table 6.2. In fact, the percentage of nonabusers with close relatives reported to be substance abusers (4%) was not appreciably lower than the percentage for decedents classified as alcoholics or narcotics abusers by physical evidence alone.

There is no reason why deceased alcoholics and narcotics abusers classified by physical evidence would be any less or more likely to have close relatives with comparable problems than would those identified by informants. However, informants who denied that decedents had a drinking or drug problem were undoubtedly more likely to deny such problems of close relatives than were informants who acknowledged decedents' alcoholism or narcotism. Thus there was evidence of much underreporting by informants in our study, not only of the decedents' problems due to alcohol or narcotics use, but also of such problems among decedents' close relatives. With this

Table 6–2. Alcohol and Narcotics Problems of Close Relatives According to Method of Classifying Decedents as Alcoholics and Narcotics Abusers

METHOD OF CLASSIFICATION OF ALCOHOLICS AND/OR NARCOTICS ABUSERS	N	PERCENTAGE WITH SUBSTANCE ABUSE REPORTED FOR CLOSE RELATIVES
Informant[a]	(724)	21.0%
Physical evidence only	(418)	6.7
Nonabusers	(812)	4.1

a. Informant admission, with or without physical evidence.

in mind, we can estimate the percentage of all alcoholics and narcotics abusers in our study who have close relatives with comparable problems at 20 percent or more (not including relatives of decedents whose drinking or drug problems were not known by informants). Our familial rates of alcoholism and narcotism would then be approximately three and ten times the estimated overall prevalence rates of 7 and 2 percent, respectively. This indicates that both conditions are familial, with some evidence presented earlier of exchangeability between these substances.

Much other evidence indicates that alcoholism is a familial disease. Goodwin has observed that "without exception, every family study of alcoholism has shown higher rates among the relatives of alcoholics than in the general population" (10). According to McCord and McCord, the percentage of sons who become alcoholics is two to three times higher if a parent is an alcoholic (11). Reporting on his own survey in America and a comparable one in Zurich, Switzerland, Bleuler concluded that alcoholism occurred much more frequently among both blood relatives and spouses of alcoholics than in the general population (12).

Interviews with first-degree relatives of alcoholics (child, sibling, or parent) have suggested that alcoholism is a familial disease associated with affective disorder (mood disturbances) in female relatives and alcoholism in male relatives (13). In our study, 61 siblings of 49 alcoholic decedents were reported to have a drinking problem; 74 percent of them were brothers. Also, recall that 79 percent of the 803 decedents classified as alcoholics were men. But as more women drink and as they drink more, a larger percentage will be at risk of becoming alcoholics.

Although less research has been done on narcotics abuse as a familial disease, the heavy concentration of young heroin addicts in urban ghetto communities and within a relatively narrow age range (14) suggests that their siblings would be very susceptible to heroin use and addiction. A study of drinking and drug problems of U.S. Army enlisted men before, during, and after service in Vietnam shows that alcohol use was their most serious drug problem before and after Vietnam service (15). During Vietnam service, however, alcohol problems decreased and opiate use increased greatly. When alcohol and opiates were equally available, these servicemen used opiates more often than alcohol. When opiates were more difficult to obtain, however, they frequently reverted to excessive alcohol use.

The patterns of multiple drug use among narcotics abusers in several studies—including our own (see Chapter 4)—indicate that a relatively large proportion have problems because of both heroin and alcohol use (16). Ten or twenty years ago at the New York City Medical Examiner's Office, almost all alcoholics had only alcohol in their tissues when they died, and dead narcotics addicts usually had only the heroin metabolite, morphine. In the heroin addict today, postmortem toxicologic evidence of methadone, barbiturates, tranquilizers, cocaine, and alcohol, in addition to or instead of heroin, may be found; and in the alcoholic, other depressants are often present, as shown in Chapter 4. These findings demonstrate the importance of availability of drugs and of cultural factors in the addict's drug of choice, weakening the idea that the addict depends on a specific substance.

Our data point to a shift in drug choice among substance abusers from alcohol to heroin over the span of one generation. Alcohol was the only drug mentioned for all but two of the nineteen parents reported to have alcohol or other drug problems whose children were classified as narcotics abusers in our sample. Similarly, alcohol was the only drug implicated for fifteen of the sixteen parents of decedents with both conditions; the latter were almost always primarily narcotics abusers rather than alcoholics. Twenty of the 32 narcotics abusers having an alcoholic parent had lived in New York City all or most of their lives. Thus the change over time in substance abuse may reflect both the availability of heroin in New York City and a generational shift away from reliance on alcohol alone. It is too early, however, to determine whether this change in drug of choice by today's addicts is more than a transient rebellion against their parents' alcoholism.

In order to determine the relative effect of heredity and environment on alcoholism and narcotism, it is necessary to examine their prevalence among paired subjects who share the same hereditary but different environmental backgrounds, or vice versa. Most children are raised by their natural parents, so that their heredity and environment derive from the same source and are inseparable in practice.

There are four usual means of circumventing this problem. Studies of (a) identical versus fraternal twins, where their environmental backgrounds are very similar, but the genetic factors differ; (b) adopted or foster children raised completely apart from their biological parents who are known either to have or not to have the condition being investigated; (c) siblings raised separately by natural parents and by adoptive or foster parents, where their heredities are similar but their environments differ; and (d) linkage between the condition under study and proven genetic traits or markers such as colorblindness (17). An important study of adopted sons comparing (a) those with and without an alcoholic biological parent and (b) those with an alcoholic parent to their nonadopted brothers has been conducted by Goodwin (10). Our data provide an indication of the extent to which alcoholism and narcotics abuse are familial conditions, but not on the relative importance of heredity and environment.

Homicide and Suicide Rates

Based on the data presented in Table 6.3, homicide and suicide, as well as alcoholism and narcotism, run in families. Suicide rates for relatives of suicide victims have been shown to be two to three times higher than those in the general population, suggesting that suicidal tendencies do run in families (18). However, a search through the literature revealed no studies on familial patterns in homicides.

There were approximately 1000 homicides and 500 suicides of persons eighteen years of age or older in the Bronx, Manhattan, Queens, or Staten Island during the twelve-month study period which began in August 1974 (19). As mentioned above, about 3,900,000 adults lived in these four boroughs, so that the annual homicide and suicide rates were roughly 0.02 and 0.01 percent, respectively. The annual rates for close relatives of homicide and suicide victims who died of the same violent causes, estimated from the percentages in Table 6.3, would be much greater than the overall rates for New York City adults, which is probably more suggestive of environmental than hereditary etiologic factors. Homicide was the most frequent mode of unnatural death among close relatives of persons in our sample followed in order by alcoholism, narcotism, and suicide. Close relatives, moreover, most often died in the same violent manner as persons in our sample.

Table 6–3. Selected Causes of Death of Persons in our Sample and Close Relatives[a]

CAUSE OF DEATH OF ONE OR MORE CLOSE RELATIVES	N:	Homicide (546)	Suicide (336)	Alco-holism[b] (310)	Narcotism[b] (247)	Both Condi-tions[b] (60)
				CAUSE OF DEATH OF PERSONS IN OUR SAMPLE		
Homicide		6.2%	2.4%	3.9%	2.4%	3.3%
Suicide		0.4	3.3	1.6	0.4	—
Alcoholism		1.6	0.9	7.4	1.6	3.3
Narcotism		0.9	1.2	0.3	2.8	5.0
No such deaths		90.8	92.2	86.8	92.8	88.4
Total		100%	100%	100%	100%	100%

a. Close relatives are parents, siblings, spouse, and children.
b. Alcoholism and/or narcotism alone or with other cause of death.

Conclusions

The rates of alcoholism and narcotism among close relatives of all substance abusers in our sample have been projected at approximately three and ten times the estimated overall prevalence rates of 7 and 2 percent, respectively, so that both may be considered familial conditions. Parents of narcotics abusers who were reported to be substance abusers in almost all cases had problems because of drinking rather than other drug use, which indicates a generational change from alcohol to heroin as the drug of choice. There is also evidence that multiple use of alcohol, narcotics, and other drugs has become much more common among substance abusers. These findings may be consequential in the early identification of vulnerable persons, and in the prevention, control, and treatment of alcoholism and narcotics abuse and their resultant problems.

References

1. N. Jolliffe and E. M. Jellinek, "Cirrhosis of the Liver," in: *Effects of Alcohol on the Individual, Vol. 1*, E. M. Jellinek, ed., New Haven: Yale University Press, 1942, pp. 273–309; R. E. Popham, "The Jellinek Alcoholism Estimation Formula and its Application to Canadian Data," *Quarterly Journal of Studies on Alcohol 17:* 1956, pp. 559–93.

2. M. B. Bailey, P. W. Haberman, and H. Alksne, "The Epidemiology of Alcoholism in an Urban Residential Area," *Quarterly Journal of Studies on Alcohol 26:* 1965, pp. 19–40.

3. M. B. Bailey, P. W. Haberman, and J. Sheinberg, "Identifying Alcoholics in Population Surveys: A Report on Reliability," *Quarterly Journal of Studies on Alcohol 27:* 1966, pp. 300–15.

4. P. W. Haberman and J. Sheinberg, "Implicative Drinkers Reported in a Household Survey," *Quarterly Journal of Studies on Alcohol 28:* 1967, pp. 538–43.

5. D. Cahalan, I. H. Cisin, and H. M. Crossley, *American Drinking Practices,* New Brunswick, N. J.: Rutgers Center of Alcohol Studies, 1969.

6. H. A. Mulford, "Drinking and Deviant Drinking, 1963," *Quarterly Journal of Studies on Alcohol 25:* 1964, pp. 634–50.

7. Second Report of the National Commission on Marijuana and Drug Abuse, *Drug Use in America: Problem in Perspective,* Washington, D.C.: U.S. Government Printing Office, 1973, p. 143.

8. *New York State Drug Abuse Program: State Plan Update,* Albany, N. Y.: New York State Office of Drug Abuse Services, July, 1977.

9. 1970 Decennial Census Data, U.S. Department of Commerce, Bureau of the Census, from the Community Council of Greater New York, Department of Research and Program Planning Information.

10. D. Goodwin, *Is Alcoholism Hereditary?,* New York: Oxford University Press, 1976, pp. 43–62.

11. W. McCord and J. McCord, *Origins of Alcoholism,* Stanford, Cal.: Stanford University Press, 1960.

12. M. Bleuler, "Familial and Personal Background of Alcoholics" and "A Comparative Study of Swiss and American Alcoholic Patients," in: *Etiology of Chronic Alcoholism,* O. Diethelm, ed., Springfield, Ill.: Charles C. Thomas, 1955, pp. 110–78.

13. G. Winokur et al., "Diagnosis and Familial Psychiatric Illness in 259 Alcoholic Probands," *Archives of General Psychiatry 23:* 1970, pp. 104–11; J. Rimmer and D. S. Chambers, "Alcoholism: Methodological Considerations in the Study of Family Illness," *American Journal of Orthopsychiatry 39:* 1969, pp. 760–68.

14. I. F. Lukoff, "Consequences of Use: Heroin and Other Narcotics," in: *Report of the Task Force on the Epidemiology of Heroin and Other Narcotics,* J. D. Rittenhouse, ed., Menlo Park, Cal.: Stanford Research Institute, 1976, pp. 119–39.

15. D. W. Goodwin, D. H. Davis, and L. N. Robins, "Drinking Amid Abundant Illicit Drugs," *Archives of General Psychiatry 32:* 1975, pp. 230–33.

16. National Clearinghouse for Drug Abuse Information, NIDA, *Polydrug Use: An Annotated Bibliography,* Washington, D. C.: DHEW Publication No. (ADM) 1975, pp. 75–225; A. Richman, G. Jackson, and H. Trigg, "Follow-up of Methadone Maintenance Patients Hospitalized for Abuse

of Alcohol and Barbiturates," in: *Fifth National Conference on Methadone Treatment, 1973 Proceedings*, R. L. Dupont and R. S. Freeman, eds., New York: NAPAN, 1973, pp. 1484–93; G. W. Jackson and A. Richman, "Alcohol Use among Narcotic Addicts," *Alcohol Health and Research World 1:* 1973, pp. 25–28.

17. R. Cruz-Coke and A. Varela, "Inheritance of Alcoholism," *Lancet 2:* Dec. 10, 1966, pp. 1282–84; A. Varela et al., "Color Vision Defects in Non-Alcoholic Relatives of Alcoholic Patients," *British Journal of Addiction 64:* 1969, pp. 67–73.

18. R. A. Blath, J. N. McClure, and R. D. Wetzel, "Familial Factors in Suicide," *Diseases of the Nervous System 34: 1973*, pp. 90–93.

19. *Vital Statistics by Health Areas and Health Center Districts, 1974*, New York City Department of Health, Bureau of Health Statistics and Analysis, 1976.

7

Implications and Recommendations

The role of alcohol and other drugs in violent deaths has been established in various studies in which data on specific relationships, such as suicide and chronic alcoholism, or the blood alcohol level of motor vehicle fatalities, from one source are utilized retrospectively. In our study, the involvement of alcohol, narcotics, and other drugs in all types of unnatural deaths is interpreted concurrently from various sources of data available for individual cases — informant statements, medical history, autopsy and toxicologic findings, and certified cause of death.

Our data delineate the use and abuse of different mood-altering drugs by adults whose deaths are unnatural. Medical examiner data such as ours also reflect the demographic characteristics of users who reside in the jurisdiction under study, and the patterns of drug use. Substance abusers whose deaths are investigated by the Medical Examiner in New York City are predominantly young Hispanic or black men. However, our findings seem to reflect a trend toward more alcohol and narcotics abuse by somewhat younger adults, women, and whites. We have also found an increase in multiple drug use: alcohol and narcotics taken together or concomitantly with other drugs. Since the 1972 pilot study (1), our more recent toxicologic findings indicate an increase in the abuse of Darvon (propoxyphene) and cocaine.

The effectiveness of drug treatment programs can also be measured in part by medical examiner data. The unnatural deaths of current or previous patients and their postmortem toxicologic findings provide a partial evaluation of major treatment efforts, such as methadone maintenance. Illicit methadone use has become widespread as methadone maintenance treatment has expanded. More deaths in New York City are now associated with methadone among both MMTP patients and nonpatients. Furthermore, despite methadone's alleged blocking effect on heroin, in 16 percent of the deaths due to narcotics use, both drugs were present in postmortem tests.

If the number of decedent abusers, their use of mood-altering substances, and their demographic characteristics can be documented, medical examiner data can then be used to reflect overall changes in (a) the prevalence of alcoholism and narcotics addiction in the study area, (b) patterns of drug use, and (c) demographic characteristics of users. For a complete understanding of changes in drug prevalence and in the characteristics of users from medical examiner data, changes in the general population of the study area must also be examined. The home addresses and places of death of alcoholics and addicts can be used to locate neighborhoods or blocks within a city which are commonly frequented by such persons.

Alcohol is usually not indicated on the death certificate as a contributing factor in accidental (or homicidal) deaths or those resulting from concomitant use of alcohol and other drugs. Similarly, other drugs are not mentioned in unnatural deaths unless such deaths were directly related to drug use, as in a suicidal or accidental overdose of pills. The standard death certificate in the United States shown here (p. 106), unfortunately, has no provision to indicate contributory alcoholism, narcotics addiction, or other drug abuse. Most tabulations are based on the single diagnostic entry selected as the underlying cause of death (2). Substance abuse as a contributory cause is infrequently and inconsistently recorded and is rarely reported except in studies such as ours.

In large measure because of the nature of the death certificate itself, present-day mortality data do not reflect the true contribution of substance abuse to unnatural death. If death certificate information alone were utilized, 54 percent of the alcohol-related deaths and 44 percent of the narcotics-related deaths in our study would have been

THE CERTIFICATE NOT VALID UNLESS FILED IN THE HEALTH DEPARTMENT
1. Typewrite or print only with black or blue-black ink.
2. Certificates containing alterations or omissions are unacceptable.
3. "Date filed." "Certificate No." and this space, reserved for Health Department use only.

CERTIFICATE OF DEATH

Certificate No. ....

Institution	
Boro-Resid.	
Area-Dist.	
R C	
Nativ. Dec.	
Cause 1	
Operation	
Att.-Autop.	
Cem.	
Type Accid.	
Occurrence	

DATE FILED

1. NAME OF DECEASED *(Type or Print)*   First Name   Middle Name   Last Name

MEDICAL CERTIFICATE OF DEATH *(To be filled in by the Physician)*

2. PLACE OF DEATH — NEW YORK CITY: a. Borough of   b. Name of Hospital or Institution. If not in hospital, street address

3a. DATE AND HOUR OF DEATH (Month) (Day) (Year)   **3b. Hour** AM / PM   **4. SEX**   **5. APPROXIMATE AGE**

6. I HEREBY CERTIFY that, in accordance with the provisions of law, I took charge of the dead body at..on................day of....................19.......
I further certify from the investigation and post mortem examination (with) (without) autopsy that in my opinion, death occurred on the date and at the hour stated above and resulted from (natural causes) (accident) (suicide) (homicide) (undetermined circumstances pending further investigation,) and that the causes of death were:

PART 1
a. Immediate cause
b. Due to or as a consequence of
c. Due to or a consequence of

PART 2 — Contributory causes

M.E. Case No.

Signed .... M.D.
(Medical Investigator) (Junior) (Assistant) (Associate) (Deputy Chief) (Chief) (Medical Examiner)

PERSONAL PARTICULARS *(To be filled in by Funeral Director)*

7. USUAL RESIDENCE — a. State   b. County   c. City or Town   d. Inside city limits of "7c" ☐ Yes ☐ No
e. Street and house number   f. Apt.   g. Length of residence or stay in City of New York immediately prior to death.

8. SINGLE, MARRIED, WIDOWED or DIVORCED (Write in word)   **9. NAME OF SURVIVING SPOUSE** (If wife, give maiden name)

10. DATE OF BIRTH OF DECEDENT (Month) (Day) (Year)   **11. AGE** at last birthday Yrs   If under year mos. days   If LESS than 1 day hrs or min.

12a. USUAL OCCUPATION (Kind of work done during most of working life, even if retired.)   b. KIND of BUSINESS or INDUSTRY   **13. SOCIAL SECURITY NO.**

14. BIRTHPLACE (State or Foreign Country)   **15. OF WHAT COUNTRY WAS DECEASED A CITIZEN AT TIME OF DEATH.**

16. ANY OTHER NAME(s) BY WHICH DECEDENT WAS KNOWN

17. NAME OF FATHER OF DECEDENT   **18. MAIDEN NAME OF MOTHER OF DECEDENT**

19a. NAME OF INFORMANT   b. RELATIONSHIP TO DECEASED   c. ADDRESS

20a. NAME OF CEMETERY OR CREMATORY   b. LOCATION (City, Town or State & Country)   c. DATE of Burial or Cremation

21a. FUNERAL DIRECTOR   b. ADDRESS

BUREAU OF VITAL RECORDS—DEPARTMENT OF HEALTH—THE CITY OF NEW YORK

16II (Rev. 7/72)
25M-702073(77)
346

overlooked. The full extent of the contribution of alcohol and other drugs to unnatural deaths during a given time period requires a study which goes beyond the tabulations of routinely reported mortality data and must include deaths which are not reported to the medical examiner. Moreover, such studies must be repeated in order to ascertain changes in substance abuse among decedents over time.

There have been some recent efforts to develop a systematic and comprehensive method of collecting and reporting drug-related deaths. Because of difficulties in postmortem evaluation of tolerance, Baden has classified the methadone users whose deaths he investigates as either tolerant (in maintenance treatment) or nontolerant. The causes of death for the two groups were categorized as being due to natural causes, trauma, or abuse of different substances, alone or concurrently. Baden concluded that adequate nationwide drug-abuse mortality data grouped in a comparable manner could produce much useful information for research, development, and program planning (3).

As traditionally categorized at the Office of Chief Medical Examiner, New York City, Lettieri has also distinguished between directly and indirectly related drug deaths (4,5). Directly related drug deaths are those which would not have occurred if the drug were not present. Indirectly related drug deaths are those in which the drug may be a necessary but not sufficient factor to explain the death (such as a fatal accident) while the victim was under the influence of drugs. Lettieri has recommended that a total, comprehensive data collection system of directly and indirectly related drug deaths be implemented nationally.

Gottschalk and his colleagues (6) have proposed that narcotics deaths be categorized in the following manner:

Drug-induced, with no other agent playing a significant role

Drug in combination with other drug(s)

Drug-related, with some pre-existing physiological condition, such as diabetes

Drug in combination with accident, homicide, or suicide

Drug in combination with a medical condition probably related to drug abuse, such as hepatitis or tetanus

In order to reduce the great underreporting in government statistics on drug- and alcohol-related deaths, we fully endorse these efforts to improve the reporting system of drug deaths and further recommend that this schema be utilized in the same manner for alcohol deaths. As a first step, we propose that all relatives or other persons making identifications be routinely asked in a uniform manner, whether the decedent had problems related to drinking or other drug use as in our study. Classification of decedents as substance abusers should be based on both informant and physical evidence, not on the certified cause of death alone, which may differ among alcoholics and narcotics abusers who are homicide, suicide, or accident victims and those whose cause of death was alcoholism and/or narcotism.

Community trends in the prevalence of alcoholism and narcotics abuse can be extrapolated from yearly changes in the number of deaths directly related to alcohol or narcotics investigated by medical examiners or coroners. However, some adjustment would have to be made for the time lag between patterns of substance abuse and their consequences before a change in prevalence is reflected in mortality data—for alcoholics more than narcotic addicts. The first evidence of liver damage in chronic alcoholics is generally preceded by at least 15 years' steady drinking (7), while addicts who die of narcotism most often have an acute fatal reaction without prior warning, usually within five to ten years after first use. Thus, changes in narcotics use are revealed in fatalities much sooner than changes in alcohol use.

It is more difficult to project rates of alcoholism and narcotics abuse from mortality data than to project trends. The relatively constant relationship between alcohol consumption and mortality from cirrhosis of the liver together with a long period of effective prohibition enabled Jellinek to develop his alcoholism estimation formula (8). Since 1960, however, it has been necessary to use population surveys to measure the prevalence of alcoholism in large communities. Using alcohol consumption data and establishing the per capita consumption for all drinkers and for alcoholics, Schmidt and de Lint have recommended another method to estimate alcoholism prevalence (9). Total consumption can generally be determined by the available government reports on overall sales of alcoholic beverages. When using such reports, Keller's admonition that "it is always dangerous to make inference about alcoholism from statistics on drinking" should be recalled (10).

Suggested methods of estimating the prevalence of narcotics abuse have relied on serum hepatitis cases (11) or deaths (4), on the number of living addicts, and on the proportion of dead addicts listed in narcotics registers (12). Estimation of the prevalence of narcotics abuse from serum hepatitis data assumes a reasonably constant relationship between this condition and intravenous injection of narcotics, similar to, although weaker than, the relationship between cirrhosis of the liver and alcoholism. At this stage, hepatitis data alone are not sufficiently conclusive to determine trends in narcotics use or related deaths, except perhaps when changes in numbers of hepatitis cases occur among those demographic subgroups most vulnerable to narcotics addiction. These data may, however, suggest changing patterns of narcotics use and provoke further investigation.

Baden has presented a formula which estimates the number of narcotics addicts from a city's narcotics register and medical examiner data which has been expanded to general use by DuPont (12). To illustrate, if there were 1000 narcotics addicts whose deaths (due to narcotism or trauma) were investigated by the medical examiners in one year, and 50 percent were known to the narcotics register, and if there were 50,000 addicts listed on the register, his estimate of the addicts in the city would be 100,000. This estimate assumes that an equal proportion (50%) of living and dead addicts are known to the register. Thus, there would be 100 living addicts for each addict who died directly or indirectly of narcotics use (100,000 divided by 1000). If only directly related narcotics deaths are available, the ratio between living and dead addicts must be changed appropriately.

This example in table form is:

ON NARCOTICS REGISTER	NUMBER OF ADDICTS	
	Medical examiner cases	*Alive*
Yes	500	50,000
No	500	50,000 (presumed)
Total	1,000[a]	100,000

a. Includes directly and indirectly related narcotics deaths.

Two means of estimating the prevalence of alcoholism and narcotics abuse are suggested by our data. First, a ratio should be calculated between prevalence estimates based on population surveys, narcotics registers, or by other means and the number of medical examiner cases classified as alcoholics or narcotics abusers by standardized informant and physical evidence in the same year. Death certificate information alone should not be used to calculate this ratio, since a substantial number of alcoholics and narcotics abusers in our study population died of some cause other than alcoholism and/or narcotism. If this ratio remains relatively constant in repeated surveys, the prevalence estimate could be subsequently projected from medical examiner data. [The Jellinek formula, it should be noted, was also compared with surveys and other independent methods of estimating alcoholism prevalence in various areas shortly after it was developed (13).]

If a survey estimate of the number of alcoholics in a large city were 200,000 and the number of medical examiner cases classified as alcoholics in the same year were 1000, the ratio of living to dead alcoholics would be 200 to one. If a second year's survey estimate of alcoholics were 250,000 and the number of medical examiner cases classified as alcoholics in the same year were 1250, the ratio would remain 200 to one. If there were 1500 medical examiner cases in a subsequent year classified as alcoholics, the projection of the estimated number of alcoholics in the city would be 300,000 (1500 multiplied by 200).

This example in table form is:

NUMBER OF ALCOHOLICS

Year	Medical examiner cases	Alive	Source
1	1,000	200,000	survey
2	1,250	250,000	survey
3	1,500	300,000	projection

It must be emphasized that subsequent prevalence projections would be no more accurate than the initial population survey or narcotics register source data. The Jellinek formula produced reasonable estimates of alcoholism prevalence in the United States only for about ten years after Prohibition was repealed. Similarly, other means of estimating prevalence may lose their validity over time. Finally, the estimated number of substance abusers will include a substantial minority—20 percent in our study—who would be classified as both alcoholics and narcotics abusers.

Another way to estimate alcoholism and narcotism prevalence would be to select a cause of death—such as homicide—in large cities with a sufficiently large number of cases each year, and to determine the prevalence of alcoholism or narcotics abuse among the victims. If the proportion of victims who were substance abusers remains about the same, relative changes in the number of alcoholics and narcotics abusers could be formulated from changes in the homicide rate. In New York City between 1972 and 1976, the number of homicide victims eighteen years of age or older has remained relatively constant—approximately 1500 annually (14). Thus, the number of substance abusers estimated in this manner would have also remained about the same during this five-year period. If the prevalence rates of alcoholism or narcotism were also estimated by an independent method in a given year, the number of alcoholics or addicts in subsequent years by the second method could be estimated from changes in the homicide rate.

In addition to the limitations of the first method of estimating prevalence suggested by our data, the second method assumes that the percentage of homicide victims who are alcoholics and/or narcotics abusers will remain unchanged—in our study, 19 percent alcoholism alone and 27 percent narcotics abuse alone or with alcoholism. Despite the drawbacks of our proposed methods, (a) the time and cost advantages and (b) the potential accuracy in estimating the prevalence of alcoholism and narcotics abuse from data regularly and uniformly collected justify further efforts to develop the use of mortality statistics for this purpose.

In conclusion, it is apparent that death certificate data are misleading in determining the true contribution of substance abuse in unnatural deaths in this country. Based on recent patterns of drug use, it appears at this time that the use of mood-altering substances, including some that have not yet been discovered, will increase in the foreseeable future. For proper program development and establishment of priorities to improve the nation's health and to prevent unnecessary death, a new standard death certificate must be utilized which will reflect the contribution of alcohol, narcotics and other drugs to the cause of death.

References

1. Study, "Alcoholism among Decedents in New York City," supported by Grant No. R01-MH20997 from the National Institute on Alcohol Abuse and Alcoholism, Paul W. Haberman, principal investigator.
2. P. W. Haberman, "The Reliability and Validity of the Data," in: *Poverty and Health: A Sociological Analysis*, J. Kosa, A. Antonovsky and I. K. Zola, eds., Cambridge, Mass.: Harvard University Press, 1969, pp. 343–83.
3. M. M. Baden and R. S. Turoff, "Deaths of Persons Using Methadone in New York City—1971," *Proceedings of Committee on Problems of Drug Dependence, National Academy of Sciences, National Research Council,* 1973, pp. 318–24.
4. D. J. Lettieri and M. S. Backenheimer, "A Step Towards Resolution of the Problem: Considerations for a Reporting System of Drug-Deaths," in: *Proceedings of Fifth National Conference on Methadone Treatment,* Washington, D.C.: National Association for the Prevention of Addiction to Narcotics, March, 1973, pp. 336–44.
5. M. M. Baden, "Narcotic Abuse: A Medical Examiner's View," *New York State Journal of Medicine 72*:1972, pp. 834–40.
6. L. A. Gottschalk and F. L. McGuire, "Psychosocial and Biomedical Aspects of Deaths Associated with Heroin and Other Narcotics," in: *Report of the Task Force on the Epidemiology of Heroin and Other Narcotics,* J. D. Rittenhouse, ed., Menlo Park, Cal.: Stanford Research Institute, 1976, pp. 77–81; L. A. Gottschalk, "Indicators of Drug Abuse—Drug-Involved Death," in: *The Epidemiology of Drug Abuse,* L. G. Richards and L. B. Blevens, eds., NIDA Research Monograph 10, Washington, D. C.: U. S. Government Printing Office, 1977, pp. 98–122.
7. S. Sherlock, *Diseases of the Liver and Biliary System,* Philadelphia: F. A. Davis, 4th Ed., 1968, pp. 412–25.
8. N. Jolliffe and E. M. Jellinek, "Cirrhosis of the Liver," in: *Effects of Alcohol on the Individual,* E. M. Jellinek, ed., Vol. I, New Haven: Yale University Press, 1942, pp. 273–309; R. E. Popham, "The Jellinek Alcoholism Estimation Formula and its Application to Canadian Data," *Quarterly Journal of Studies on Alcohol 17*:1956, pp. 559–93.
9. W. Schmidt and J. de Lint, "Estimating the Prevalence of Alcoholism from Alcohol Consumption and Mortality Data," *Quarterly Journal of Studies on Alcohol 31*:1970, pp. 957–64.

10. M. Keller, "The Definition of Alcoholism and the Estimation of its Prevalence," in: *Society, Culture and Drinking Patterns*, D. J. Pittman and C. R. Snyder, eds., New York: Wiley, 1962, pp. 310–29.

11. M. Alexander, "Indicators of Drug Abuse—Hepatitis," *The Epidemiology of Drug Abuse*, L. G. Richards and L. B. Blevens, eds., NIDA Research Monograph 10, Washington, D.C.: U.S. Government Printing Office, 1977; pp. 123–29.

12. R. L. Dupont and R. M. Katon, "Development of a Heroin-Addiction Treatment Program, "*Journal of American Medical Association 216:* May 24, 1971, pp. 1320–24; R. L. Dupont, "Profile of a Heroin-Addiction Epidemic," *New England Journal of Medicine 285:* August 5, 1971, pp. 320–24.

13. R. E. Popham, "The Jellinek Alcoholism Estimation Formula and its Application to Canadian Data," *Quarterly Journal of Studies on Alcohol 17:* 1956, pp. 559–93.

14. Data obtained from Crime Analysis Section, New York City Police Department, June, 1977:

Appendices

Appendix A

Questionnaire for Informant Identification of Decedent

ITEM	QUESTION OR DESCRIPTION	RESPONSE PERCENTAGES
1. Borough of Death	Manhattan	55.3%
	Bronx	23.9
	Queens	19.0
	Staten Island	1.8
	Total	100%
2. Informant	Relationship of primary informant to *decedent*	
	Spouse	13.8%
	Brother	17.7
	Sister	10.3
	Father	9.4
	Mother	7.6
	Son	6.7
	Daughter	2.9
	Other relative	19.7
	Friend	10.4
	Other	1.5
	Total	100%
3. Last time informant and decedent spoke	When was the last (most recent) time you spoke to *the decedent*?	
	Within one day prior to death	37.0%

ITEM	QUESTION OR DESCRIPTION	RESPONSE PERCENTAGES
	Within one week prior to death	30.8
	Within one month prior to death	17.8
	Within six months prior to death	9.6
	One year or more prior to death	4.9
	Total	100%
3A. Decedent/informant in same household	If spoke within one month prior to death and applicable: Did *the decedent* live in the same household with you?	
	No	71.1%
	Yes	28.9
	Total	100%
4. Sex	Male	76.2%
	Female	23.8
	Total	100%
5. Birthplace	Where was *the decedent* born? U.S. state; or foreign country.	
	United States	(70.2%)
	New York City	39.7%
	Northeast	7.5
	South	19.7
	Elsewhere in U.S.	3.3
	Puerto Rico	13.5
	Other Western Hemisphere— English speaking	1.5
	Dominican Republic	1.4
	Cuba	1.0
	Other Western Hemisphere—not English speaking	2.4
	Europe	(8.0)
	Ireland	1.3
	Germany/Austria	1.3
	Italy	1.1
	Eastern Europe	2.9
	Elsewhere in Europe	1.4
	Asia, Africa, Australia	1.1
	Unknown	1.0
	Total	100%
6. Ethnicity	Hispanic	20.9%
	White	41.2
	Black	37.2

ITEM	QUESTION OR DESCRIPTION	RESPONSE PERCENTAGES
	Oriental	0.7
	Total	100%
7. Age	Age at last birthday	
	18–24	18.3%
	25–29	15.3
	30–34	12.4
	35–39	10.4
	40–49	17.1
	50–59	12.0
	60–69	7.9
	70–99	6.8
	Total	100%
8. Marital Status	Single	42.1%
	Married: legal	25.5
	Married: common-law	3.4
	Separated	11.9
	Divorced	8.7
	Widowed	7.7
	Unknown	0.7
	Total	100%
9. Usual occupation	What kind of work did *the decedent* usually do (before retirement)?	
	Professional, technical, managerial, or administrative workers	9.4%
	Clerical or sales workers	16.3
	Craftsmen, foremen	7.5
	Operatives	14.9
	Service workers (including 1.1% private household workers)	18.0
	Laborers	7.2
	"Odd jobs"	5.4
	Homemakers	7.4
	Students	3.3
	Service, armed forces	0.8
	Disabled, ill	1.4
	None, nothing	3.9
	Criminal/illegal occupation	0.6
	Unknown	3.8
	Total	100%
10. Place of residence	Manhattan	46.4%
	Bronx	24.7%
	Queens	16.5

ITEM	QUESTION OR DESCRIPTION	RESPONSE PERCENTAGES
	Brooklyn	4.6
	Richmond (Staten Island)	1.6
	Elsewhere in New York State/New Jersey	4.1
	Elsewhere (including 0.6% unknown)	2.2
	Total	100%
11. Health District of Residence	Street address	
12. Time in N.Y.C.	How long did *the decedent* live in New York City (years)?	
	Nonresident	5.7%
	Less than 1 year	1.8
	1–5 years	6.9
	6–9 years	5.4
	10–19 years	13.0
	20 years or more	29.7
	Entire life	36.6
	Unknown	0.8
	Total	100%
13. Principal activity	What was *the decedent* doing most of the past year—working, or something else?	
	Working	40.7%
	Looking for work, laid off	4.8
	Keeping house	8.4
	Retired	7.4%
	Going to school	3.7
	Sick	16.0
	Nothing	7.8
	Taking drugs	2.7
	Drinking	2.2
	Jail	1.0
	Service, armed forces	0.5
	Unknown, no answer	4.9
	Total	100%
14. U.S. armed forces service	Did *the decedent* ever serve in the armed forces of the U.S.? IF YES: When?	
	Males	
	Vietnam War	4.8%
	Other service	10.3
	No service	57.4
	Not asked	3.8
	Females (not asked)	23.8
	Total	100%

ITEM	QUESTION OR DESCRIPTION	RESPONSE PERCENTAGES
15. Religion	What was the religion of *the decedent* (at the time of death)?	
	Catholic	47.1%
	Protestant	37.2
	Jewish	8.5
	Other	2.5
	None	2.8
	Unknown	1.9
	Total	100%
16. Education	What was the highest grade in school that *the decedent* completed? IF APPLICABLE: Did *the decedent* graduate grade school (high school, college)?	
	None or some grade school (1–7 years)	9.9%
	Grade school graduate (8 years)	8.6
	Some high school (9–11 years)	27.3
	High school graduate (12 years)	27.4
	Some college (13–15 years)	9.3
	College graduate (16 years)	5.3
	Postgraduate work (17 years or more)	2.1
	Unknown	10.0
	Total	100%
17. Health or other problem(s) due to drinking	Did *the decedent ever* have any health problems because of drinking (alcoholic beverages)? Did *the decedent ever* have any family, money, job, or other problems because of drinking?	
	No drinking-related problems	61.0%
	Health problems	18.0
	Family problems	7.6
	Job problems	6.5
	Psychological problems	5.6
	Money problems	5.0
	Problems unspecified	0.9
	Heavy drinking only	12.2
	Unknown, no answer	4.0
	Total	121%[a]

		RESPONSE
ITEM	QUESTION OR DESCRIPTION	PERCENTAGES

17A. Last time drinking problems

IF ANY PROBLEMS DUE TO DRINKING: When was the last (most recent) time *the decedent* had any problems due to drinking (year)?

1950–69	0.2%
1970–72	0.2
1973–75	21.1
Unknown, no answer	1.3
Not asked	77.2
Total	100%

17B. Help

Did *the decedent* ever try to get help about this? IF YES: Where did *the decedent* go for help?

No help	12.0%
Hospital	4.6
Alcoholics Anonymous (AA)	2.5
Psychiatrist/psychologist	0.8
Other physician	0.4
Social agency	0.7
Clergyman	0.2
Yes, place unknown or numerous places unspecified	1.0
Unknown, no answer	1.9%
Not asked	77.2
Total	101%[a]

17C. Last time help

IF HELP: When was the last (most recent) time *the decedent* tried to get help (year)?

1950–69	0.5%
1970–72	0.5
1973–75	7.2
Unknown, no answer	0.9
Not asked	91.0
Total	100%

18. Hospitalization for liver trouble

Was *the decedent* ever hospitalized for liver trouble?

No	78.1%
Yes, for liver trouble (probably due to alcoholism)	6.1
Yes, for hepatitis, not due to alcohol use (probably related to narcotics use)	4.1
Unknown, no answer	11.7
Total	100%

		RESPONSE
ITEM	QUESTION OR DESCRIPTION	PERCENTAGES

ITEM	QUESTION OR DESCRIPTION	RESPONSE PERCENTAGES
18A. Last time hospitalization for liver trouble	IF YES: When was the last (most recent) time *the decedent* was hospitalized for that condition (year)?	
	1950–69	2.3%
	1970–72	2.0
	1973–75	5.1
	Unknown	0.8
	Not asked	89.8
	Total	100%
19. Problems due to drug use	Did *the decedent* ever have any problems because of drug use? IF YES: What drug(s) did the decedent use?	
	None	63.9%
	Heroin (morphine)	20.2
	Barbiturates/downs	5.8
	Methadone[b]	0.3[b]
	Other	4.7
	Specific drug(s) unknown	3.2
	Unknown, no answer	10.3
	Total	108%[a]
19A. If narcotics or methadone used	Was *the decedent* in a methadone maintenance program?[c]	
	Yes	13.8%
	No	6.6
	Not asked	79.6
	Total	100%
19B. Last time problems due to drug use	IF YES: When was the last (most recent) time *the decedent* had any problems due to drugs (year)?	
	1950–69	0.2%
	1970–72	1.4
	1973–75	11.7
	Unknown	12.6
	Not asked	74.2
	Total	100%
20. Cause of death of immediate family members	Do you know the cause of death of any members of *the decedent's* immediate family—his/her parents, any brother(s) or sister(s), husband/wife, or children? (Who was that? What was the cause of death?)	

ITEM	QUESTION OR DESCRIPTION	RESPONSE PERCENTAGES
	Unnatural cause of death	
	Accident	
	Motor Vehicle	2.8%
	Other	3.9
	Homicide	3.5
	Suicide	1.1
	Alcoholism	2.4
	Narcotism	1.1
	War, concentration camp	1.6
	No unnatural cause of death	83.6
	Total	100%
21. Drinking or drug problems of immediate family members	Do you know if any members of *the decedent's* immediate family ever had any problem because of drinking (alcoholic beverages) or using drugs? (Who was that? Was the problem because of alcohol, narcotics, or other drugs?)	
	Relationship	
	Brother/sister	7.0%
	Father	3.6
	Mother	1.7
	Spouse	0.5
	Child	0.2
	None	89.3
	Total	102%[a]
	Problem because of:	
	Alcohol	7.7%
	Narcotics	3.9
	Other drug(s)	0.2
	None	89.3
	Total	101%[a]
22. Interviewer appraisal of respondent's answers to questions about drinking and other drug problems	Reliable and knowledgeable	21.6%
	Reliable, but uncertain knowledge	
	Current	17.7
	Past	3.2
	Current and past	18.9
	Knowledgeable, but uncertain reliability	8.2
	Uncertain reliability and knowledge	
	Current	6.0
	Current and past	24.4
	Total	100%

ITEM	QUESTION OR DESCRIPTION	RESPONSE PERCENTAGES
23. Interviewer	Eileen Schuster	63.2%
	Betsy Feldman	36.8
	Total	100%

a. Total is greater than 100% because more than one answer was applicable in some cases.

b. Excludes all use by MMTP patients; consists of illicit use by nonpatients only.

c. Questionable MMTP status verified by Methadone Maintenance Evaluation Unit, Columbia University School of Public Health.

Appendix B

Office of Chief Medical Examiner Physical Findings Form

ITEM	DESCRIPTION	RESPONSE PERCENTAGES
1. Date of death	(month)	
	January	9.2%
	February	8.1
	March	9.2
	April	7.9
	May	8.4
	June	8.9
	July	8.8
	August	9.7
	September	8.2
	October	7.9
	November	7.0
	December	6.8
	Total	100%
2. Place of death	Name of hospital, institution, else-where, or home address	
	Hospital	45.4%
	Home	30.6
	Other residential address	7.3
	Street	8.0
	Motor vehicle	2.6
	Water	2.0
	Business address	1.6
	Subway or train	1.3
	Other	1.2
	Total	100%
3. Evidence of drinking at scene of death	Not available	24.4%
	No evidence of drinking	71.9
	Empty liquor bottles or other evidence of drinking	3.7
	Total	100%
4. Cause-of-death classification	Homicide	(27.8%)
	Shooting	14.3
	Stabbing	7.2
	Assault	4.0
	During commission of crime	1.2
	Motor vehicle accident	(10.5)
	Pedestrian	5.0
	Driver	3.8
	Passenger	1.7

ITEM	QUESTION OR DESCRIPTION	RESPONSE PERCENTAGES
	Other accident	(9.4)
	Fall	4.7
	Fire	2.3
	Drowning	1.1
	Other	1.3
	Suicide	(17.2)
	Jumping	5.6
	Pills	4.9
	Shooting	2.3
	Hanging	1.4
	Subway or train	1.0
	Other	2.0
	Natural	(2.9)
	Cardiovascular disease	1.9
	Other	1.0
	Alcoholism	(15.9)
	Alone	11.0
	With natural or accidental cause	4.9
	Narcotism	(12.7)
	Alone	9.9
	With natural or accidental cause	2.8
	Narcotism and alcoholism	(3.1)
	Alone	2.3
	With natural or accidental cause	0.8
	Acute (accidental) drug poisoning, without narcotics or alcohol	0.6
	Total	100%
5. Type of examination	Autopsy—Medical Examiner's Office (including 3.0% without examination of liver because of decomposition, coma, or damage to body)	74.9%
	Autopsy—hospital	0.4
	Incision	(11.6)
	Abdominal	10.2
	Cranial	1.0
	Abdominal and cranial	0.4
	External (including 1.8% with possible evidence of alcoholism)	13.2
	Total	100%
6. Autopsy findings	Not obtained	16.4%
	No evidence of alcoholism	44.5
	Possible evidence of alcoholism	
	Liver abnormalities	
	Fatty change—mild	9.0
	Fatty change—moderate	13.5

ITEM	QUESTION OR DESCRIPTION	RESPONSE PERCENTAGES
	Fatty change — severe	6.2
	Cirrhosis	10.0
	Hepatic failure	1.4
	Yellow jaundice	1.2
	Pancreatitis	1.1
	Ascites	1.0
	Ruptured esophageal varices	0.5
	Total	105%[a]
7. Blood or brain alcohol concentration (BAC)	Not obtained	27.0%
	Alcohol absent	43.2
	BAC	
	.01 – .04	5.3
	.05 – .09	6.3
	.10 – .14	6.0
	.15 – .19	5.3
	.20 – .29	4.9
	.30 – .39	1.4
	.40 or more	0.6
	Total	100%
8. Other chemical findings (drugs)	Not obtained	26.9%
	No other chemicals (including 0.6% with other indication of drug ingestion)	37.7
	Methadone	12.3
	Heroin or morphine (including 0.8% with quinine or lidocaine only, but heroin implicated)	9.3
	Tranquilizers	9.0
	Sedatives (mostly barbiturates; including hypnotics)	8.4
	Darvon (propoxyphene)	2.9
	Cocaine	0.7
	Carbon monoxide only	2.2
	Quinine only, alcohol implicated	0.4
	Other — prescription drugs unrelated to abuse or to cause of death, and nonprescription drugs	2.5
	Total	112%[a]
9. "Back-of-certificate narcotism"	"Back-of-certificate narcotism"	
	Alone	0.4%
	With informant and/or physical classification of narcotics abusers	1.6
	Not recorded	98.0
	Total	100%

a. Total is greater than 100% because more than one answer was applicable in some cases.

Appendix C

Approximate Percentage Differences Between Subgroups Significant at 5 Percent Level of Significance[a]

N_1	N_2	$P_1 = 10\%$ $P_1 - P_2$	$P_1 = 20\%$ $P_1 - P_2$	$P_1 = 35\%$ $P_1 - P_2$
100	100	9%	11%	14%
	200	7	10	12
	300	7	9	12
	500	7	9	11
	700	6	9	11
200	200	6	8	10
	300	6	7	9
	500	5	7	8
	700	5	6	8
	1000	5	6	8
300	300	5	7	8
	500	4	6	7
	700	4	6	7
	1000	4	5	7
	1500	4	5	6
500	500	4	5	6
	700	4	5	6
	1000	3	4	6
	1500	3	4	5
700	700	3	4	5
	1000	3	4	5
	1500	3	4	5
1000	1000	3	4	5

a. Based on the sampling errors of simple random samples. This table can be used to determine subgroup sizes necessary for percentage difference to be significant at 5% level (see *procedures* below). Adapted from table in J. Elinson, P. W. Haberman, and C. Gell, *Community Fact Book for Washington Heights, New York City, 1965–1966 and 1960–1961*, New York: Columbia University School of Public Health, 1968, pp. 100–02.

Procedures for using Appendix C

1. Find the point in the table closest to the Ns of the two subgroups to be compared.
2. Select the P_1 in the table closest to the N_1 subgroup percentage.
3. If the percentage difference, $P_1 - P_2$, at the intersection of N_1, N_2, and P_1 is *equal* to or *less* than the difference between the two subgroup percentages, they *are* significantly different.

4. If the percentage difference, $P_1 - P_2$, at the intersection of N_1, N_2, and P_1 is *greater* than the difference between the two subgroup percentages, they *are not* significantly different.

Example: From Table 4.6

ETHNICITY	ALCOHOLICS	NARCOTICS ABUSERS
	N: (581)	(339)
Hispanic	18.4%	21.8%
White	42.6	32.8

If $N_1 = 300$, $N_2 = 500$, and $P_1 = 20\%$, $P_1 - P_2$ must be at least 6% for a significant difference at the 5% level. Therefore, the difference of 3.4% (21.8% − 18.4%) between narcotics abusers and alcoholics in the percents who were Hispanic *is not* significant.

If $N_1 = 300$, $N_2 = 500$, and $P_1 = 35\%$, $P_1 - P_2$ must be at least 7% for a significant difference at the 5% level. Therefore, the difference of 9.8% (42.6% − 32.8%) between narcotics abusers and alcoholics in the percents who were white *is* significant.

Author Index

References appear at the end of each chapter (see italic page numbers in this index).

Subject Index

DATE DUE